Performance Nutritionist Faisal Alshawa supports vibrant health for busy people across the MENA region. Originally enrolled to study economics, Faisal soon changed career pathways and graduated with a Bachelors in Kinesiology from the University of Maryland and a Masters in Sports and Exercise from Loughborough University. Achieving his ultimate dream, working in football, Faisal moved to Qatar in 2014 to work in the Aspetar Sports Medicine Hospital and Aspire Academy. He was the dedicated sports nutritionist for the U-23, U-19, and U-17 Qatar National Football teams.

Professional, world-class athletes apply discipline, passion, and commitment. The expertise Faisal mastered from working with them forms the basis of how he works with people in transforming their exhaustion to vitality.

Faisal knows what it takes to make real, lasting change. In a field overloaded with health information, he's passionate about evidence-based science. He doesn't follow trends or fad diets, nor does he preach them. Because holistic health focuses on the mind, body, and spirit, it never can be a one-size-fits-all. Health is individual – starting with mindset first.

To my family, Rashad, Mona, Bader, and Nasser—thank you for being my inspiration and motivation. If it weren't for your continued love and support, I would not have been able to write my books and be where I am today.
I love you all.

Faisal Alshawa

The Lifestyle Diet

Don't Diet. Make it a Lifestyle.

AUSTIN MACAULEY PUBLISHERS™
LONDON • CAMBRIDGE • NEW YORK • SHARJAH

Copyright © Faisal Alshawa 2023

The right of Faisal Alshawa to be identified as author of this work has been asserted by the author in accordance with Federal Law No. (7) of UAE, Year 2002, Concerning Copyrights and Neighboring Rights.

All rights reserved. No part of this publication may be reproduced, stored in a retrieval system, or transmitted in any form or by any means, electronic, mechanical, photocopying, recording, or otherwise, without the prior permission of the publishers.

Any person who commits any unauthorized act in relation to this publication may be liable to legal prosecution and civil claims for damages.

The age group that matches the content of the books has been classified according to the age classification system issued by the Ministry of Culture and Youth.

ISBN – 9789948790563 – (Paperback)
ISBN – 9789948790570 – (E-Book)

Application Number: MC-10-01-6852768
Age Classification: E

First Published 2023
AUSTIN MACAULEY PUBLISHERS FZE
Sharjah Publishing City
P.O Box [519201]
Sharjah, UAE
www.austinmacauley.ae
+971 655 95 202

Introduction
Block Out the Noise

Today, we live in a world of abundance, from the number of shows and movies available on Netflix, the endless list of products we can purchase on Amazon to the many, many blogs and social media accounts providing us with nutrition information.

What should you eat? What is the best diet? What will help you lose weight?

The volume of available nutrition information is good if you can filter it correctly. The problem is that the abundance of conflicting information has confused and frustrated us more than ever before regarding what, how, and why we should be eating.

When I entered the health and nutrition field in 2008, the awareness of living healthy lifestyle was in its infancy. There weren't as many healthy restaurants or gyms as there are today, and the idea of 'clean eating' was almost non-existent. At the time, Facebook was the only social media platform I used, and the number of nutrition accounts and so-called 'influencers' were minimal. But over the years, the movement started picking up, and people became more and more health conscious.

I loved it. I loved seeing people finally appreciating this lifestyle and pushing forward to be the best and healthiest version of themselves.

But something else started to happen.

Institutes and organizations started commercializing certification programs, allowing anyone to be certified as a personal trainer, health coach, or nutritionist – without the need of a formal education degree in the field (i.e., bachelors in dietetics, physiology, sports science, or any other related field). I have tremendous respect and appreciation for those who have come to realize their passion. More importantly, they have taken a leap of courage to switch careers midway in their lives; it is a tough decision to make – so all power to them. Yet, dealing with someone's health requires a formal degree entailing years of studying and practical experience. Can we become lawyers in six months? Can we become a dentist in three months? Absolutely not. But the commercialization of certification programs has allowed any individual, irrespective of their background, to start a business and advise people, personally or through a social media account, on their *health*.

What's more? This new trend of becoming a social media 'influencer' was created. We now have individuals suddenly becoming famous in the world of social media, which is nothing more than a bubble. The scary part is that influencers are starting to *influence* and advise people on their mental, physical, and emotional health. More and more people are beginning to live what they believe to be a healthy lifestyle, not because they love it, but because they need to appear trendy and hip. They tend to follow the next overhyped health trend before moving on to the next one. They simply follow the latest trend to keep up appearances on social media. Today, people listen to people, and influencers need to be wary of their unsubstantiated information. Others will copy what they do – which can be associated with many adverse health consequences.

In addition to the excess noise from social media and some influencers, the diet culture has created a negative stigma around food. It has made us associate food with restriction, limitation, a lack of enjoyment, and less of everything – less food, fewer meals, and fewer calories.

What is diet culture anyway? According to Christy Harrison, author of *Anti-Diet*, diet culture is 'a set of beliefs that worships thinness and equates it with health and moral virtue.' The diet culture places thinness as the pinnacle of being healthy and having a healthy body. Judith Matz, therapist and author of *The Body Positivity Card Deck,* says, "In diet culture, there is a conferred status to people who are thinner, and it assumes that eating in a certain way will result in the right body size – the 'correct' body size – and good health and that it's attainable for anybody who has the 'right' willpower, the 'right' determination."

The diet culture makes us feel bad, shameful, and guilty of our food choices whenever we indulge in foods we enjoy. It associates health with thinness and thinness with good, making us judge ourselves and judge others. Concepts like this are harmful and can lead to disordered eating, obsessive behavior, food restrictions, and following fad diets to achieve the desire of being thin.

Regarding weight loss, the diet culture makes us want to be thinner regardless of the associated mental, physical, and emotional costs. It imposes the idea that losing weight will help us feel and look better. It promotes weight loss as a way to attain a higher status, making many people spend a lot of time, money and energy on becoming thinner – even though research suggests it is challenging to achieve an ideal weight and maintain it for an extended period.

There is no 'right' body size or body weight, and even if there was an 'ideal' weight or body size, it's not easy to achieve even by doing the right thing consistently. A study analyzed the data of 76,704 obese men and 99,791 obese women aged 20 years or older between 2004 and 2014 and found a 98% failure rate of diets.[18] More specifically, the 9-year follow-up period showed that 1,283 men and 2,245 women attained normal body weight. For simple obesity (body mass index = 30.0–34.9 kg/m^2), the yearly probability of getting to normal weight was one in 210 for men and one in 124 for women. For those morbidly obese (body mass index = 40.0–44.9 kg/m(2)), the probability of attaining normal weight decreased to one in 1,290 for men and one in 677 for women.[18]

We're all victims of the diet culture. In the past, I have tried the keto diet and intermittent fasting to understand what it feels like to be on a diet. I'm sure you've tried a diet, or maybe you're currently following one. We're merely doing what we've always been told to do to improve our health, well-being, and looks – which is to diet.

As a nutritionist with ten years of working experience after gaining a bachelor's degree in kinesiology, a master's degree in sports and exercise science, working with elite athletes, and helping hundreds of individuals live a healthier and happier lifestyle, I'm writing this book to convince you, through providing evidence from studies, why diets don't work for weight loss.

Disclaimer: I'll be analyzing diets through the lens of *weight loss*. Throughout this book, anything I talk about regarding dieting revolves around losing weight in a clinically healthy population and not diets to combat a medical or clinical issue; some diets are helpful for certain medical conditions.

The Lifestyle Diet will help you understand why you should ultimately prioritize your health and well-being as a *lifestyle*! I'll begin by helping you understand the history of dieting and the many diets created before diving deeper into some of today's most popular diets. These include the ketogenic diet, plant-based diets, the paleo diet, detox diets, and intermittent fasting. After reviewing these diets and providing further input from experts in the industry, I'll help you make healthy eating a lifestyle. By the end of this book, you'll never need to diet again!

I want to help ease your mind and reduce the stress, frustration, and confusion of this daily information overload. This is your opportunity to understand things from a qualified and experienced nutritionist who has never advocated any diet to anyone yet has achieved positive results with hundreds of clients through an anti-dieting approach.

After all, to live your best and healthiest life for the long term requires you to focus on making habitual and behavioral changes to how you eat. Lifestyle eating means taking small and incremental steps every day to continually improve yourself and develop positive habits which will stick with you for the long haul. Diets provide a quick fix to a long-life problem experienced by many people; it is a short-term solution. To truly make healthy eating a lifestyle, you have to implement healthy practices every day, of every week, of every month of every year of your life. That's what lifestyle actually means. *The Lifestyle Diet* will help you get there.

For those who read my first book, *Fill Your Mind Before You Fill Your Plate*, you know that mindfulness is one of the five pillars of living a healthier lifestyle. Well, here's your chance to be mindful. Here's your chance to stay in the zone while you acquire science-based information on why diets don't work.

Block out the noise brought to you by unqualified people and the diet culture.

Section 1
Diets Don't Work

"I never worry about diets. The only carrots that interest me are the number you get in a diamond."
—Mae West

Chapter 1
The History of Dieting

According to the Cambridge English Dictionary, a diet means 'the food or drink usually eaten by a person or group.' A diet is the accumulation of food we consume, which varies in kind, shape, and form.

Cavemen were the first to get into this whole eating thing – but they didn't care about what they ate or how they looked – they just ate what they had. It turns out that our deep desire and obsession with dieting and weight loss dates back 150 years.

The word diet stems from the Greek word 'diatia,' which refers to a way of living whereby we focus on self-control and eating a balanced and moderate amount.

The days of dieting and eating well started with the early Greeks, around 400 BC. Have you ever wondered why all Greek statues depicting Gods and Goddesses (and other individuals) have such amazing bodies? All of them carved to perfection, showing their muscular, lean physique with six-pack abs.

It's because a healthy body represents a healthy mind and a healthy life. If you looked like a healthy person with a healthy body, then you were someone who looked like a

Greek God—and how amazing does that feel? Greeks idealized muscular and lean bodies, not like today's obsession with being 'skinny'.

The Greeks were hugely into fitness. Wealthy individuals with a lot of free time used to train up to eight hours a day, naked, of course. In addition, they held many beauty contests for women, which required plenty of exercise and dieting.

Hippocrates, a Greek physician, had his ideas about dieting. He believed fat people suffered from pain, aches, poor sleep, constipation, and other issues simply because of what and how much they ate. So he recommended strict dieting, an exercise regimen, and, unfortunately, vomiting.

Then came the early Christians between 600–1000 AD. It was during this period that people starved themselves as an act of holiness. St. Augustine, St. Anthony, and others treated their bodies poorly and starved themselves, frequently leading to hallucinations resulting from anorexia mirabilis or what was considered 'holy anorexia.'

In 1066 AD, William the Conqueror introduced the liquid diet. He ate so much and grew so fat that once he tried to mount his horse, he fell off and hit the ground headfirst. Embarrassed, he pretended he was kissing the ground. After this moment, he went on a liquid diet, but not your modern-day juice cleanse or water fast – he went on a strict alcohol-only diet. Unfortunately, the next time he attempted to mount his horse, he fell off, and the saddle cut through his gut. He died. He was so overweight that when priests put him into a coffin, his intestines burst open.

Fast-forward to 1500 AD, the Renaissance began as well as the renaissance of dieting. People started to care more about being sexy and secular. It was frowned upon to be overweight since there was not much left to eat, so being overweight was considered immoral – people thought such individuals were eating all their food. Kim Kardashian and other celebrities are now bringing back 'waist training corsets,' which started during the Renaissance. During this time, women began wearing corsets to make them appear slimmer – not wanting to go through the effort of dieting. Little did they know such corsets cut into their skin, eventually causing wounds that got infected and led to death.

In 1558, the world's first diet book, *The Art of Living Long*, was published by Luigi Cornaro. Cornaro was an overweight Italian who, at the age of 40, realized that being overweight caused many issues he was tired of facing. Exhausted from feeling and living this way, he adopted a diet similar to obese and anorexic individuals and lived off 350 grams of food and 414ml of wine. In his book, Cornaro advised people to live the same way. He lived to almost 100, and in the last years of his life, he only ate egg yolks.

In the 1600s, there was a shift to a more Mediterranean style diet. Italian author Giacomo Castelvetro wrote *The Fruits, Herbs, and Vegetables of Italy*. He promoted more of an Italian way of eating, focusing on fruits, fresh vegetables, and oils like olive oil. Unfortunately, during this time, there began an extreme shortage of food in Europe. So people used to eat potatoes as a way to suppress their appetite. In one instance, starving cartoonists called George IV the 'Prince of Whales.'

During the 1700s, many individuals, including famous ones, struggled with being overweight, and experienced common symptoms like bloating and constipation. They wondered why thin people can eat so much and not gain weight, while others could eat less yet still gain weight. Samuel Jackson, an English writer who made significant contributions to English literature, was one of those people, but he admittedly consumed excess food.

Dr. George Cheyne, a mathematician, philosopher, and physician, published books like *An Essay on Health and Long Life* and *The Natural Method of Curing the Disease of the Body*, which advocated the health benefits of a vegetarian diet and brought vegetarianism to life. Dr. Cheyne was overweight, so he went on a diet of milk and vegetables but regained all the weight once he started eating regular foods again.

In 1860, William Banting, an English undertaker, began to popularize the idea of going on a low carbohydrate diet. His was the first diet that went full-fledged and appealed to the masses.

Banting wasn't a scientist, but he was obese. As a result, he suffered from some health issues and even began to lose his sight and became increasingly deaf. A doctor advised him to start exercising more, but he found that exercise increased his appetite and ate even more. Banting tried several diets, including starvation, but ended up in hospital.

When Banting met Dr. William Harvey, an ENT (ear, nose, and throat) specialist, he advised him to give up all foods containing sugar and starch such as bread, butter, milk, sugar, beer, and potatoes. After a few months of following this regime, Banting lost weight, and impressively, his sight and hearing returned to normal.

Throughout his experience, he wrote a personal testimonial known as *The Letter on Corpulence, Addressed to the Public.* Through this letter, which became a self-published book, the Banting Diet came to life – essentially highlighting the benefits of a low carbohydrate diet.

In the 1820s, an English poet, Lord Byron, a founding father of the Romantic movement, was arguably one of the sexiest men of his time. Naturally, everyone wanted to look like him. He faced the issue of easy and rapid weight gain, so he had to starve himself to keep looking slim and sexy. It was the beginning of the Apple Cider Vinegar Diet, where you add one tablespoon of apple cider vinegar to a glass of water and drink it before every meal. Lord Byron used to drench a lot of his food in vinegar.

Fun fact: In 1899, Dr. Howard Kelly performed the first tummy tuck at the Johns Hopkins Hospital, where he removed 15 pounds of fat from a patient's belly.

Now we head into the 1900s. This period saw the start of arguably one of the most random and weirdest diets known as 'Fletcherism.' Howard Fletcher created this diet as he was unfortunately too fat to qualify for health insurance. He derived this from the idea of chewing your food 32 times and only swallowing what naturally slipped down your throat before spitting out the rest. He eventually refined this to chewing your food until it was almost liquid, or chewing it 100 times, before swallowing.

Fun fact: Those who followed the 'Fletcher Method' were known as 'Fletchers.' Some famous people, including John D. Rockefeller and John Kelloggs (founder of the cereal brand, Kelloggs), advocated this diet.

It was during this time that Dr. Lulu Hunt Peters published the first calorie-counting book. The American doctor's bestselling diet book, *Dieting and Health: With Key to the Calories,* sold over two million copies. She was known as the 'queen of calories' since she introduced the world to the idea of counting calories.

By trying different things, gaining knowledge while earning her medical degree at the University of California, and researching, she concluded that weight loss is achieved when one burns more calories than consumed. It still holds, which is indeed a fundamental behind weight and fat loss. No special diet is needed. Simply put your body in a calorie deficit (burning more calories than you consume), and you will lose weight and fat.

Fun fact: Dr. Lulu devised an accurate way to count calories in food and help people understand their ideal calorie consumption for their weight.

From this point, science and research regarding dieting began to emerge faster than ever before. Below is a brief timeline of diets that appeared after this:

1920: The Keto Diet

This diet is based on the consumption of high-fat and low-carb foods, consuming 75% of your caloric intake from fats and less than 50 grams (some studies suggest less than 20 grams) of carbohydrates per day. The diet initially emerged as a way to help with epilepsy and other health issues.

1925: The Lucky Strike Diet

Lucky Strike is a tobacco company. The popularity of smoking coupled with the increased desire to look slim led Lucky Strike to promote smoking cigarettes to suppress appetite. Their motto was 'Reach for a Lucky, instead of a sweet.'

The 1930s: Macrobiotic Diet

A diet focused heavily on improving gut health by consuming organic and locally grown produce such as whole grains, fruits, vegetables, and legumes.

The 1940s: Mediterranean Diet

The Mediterranean Diet varies depending on the country and region. It's about following the diet of Mediterranean countries composed of vegetables, fruits, legumes, pulses, grains, and healthy fats like fish and olive oil.

Honestly, of all diets, this is the only one that resonates with me. It's an excellent way to eat.

1941: The Lemonade Diet

Otherwise known as the Master Cleanse Diet, the lemonade diet is about drinking a mixture of lemon, maple syrup, cayenne pepper, and water six times a day for ten days straight. Beyoncé was once an advocate of this diet, losing around 20 pounds in two weeks to prepare for the Coachella Music Festival show.

Don't get inspired by this; you'll soon find out why this is terrible for you. Just because Beyoncé did it and lost weight doesn't mean you will.

1944: Veganism

Donald Watson coined the word 'vegan' and ultimately led to the vegan diet we know today. After becoming a vegetarian after the age of 14, he gathered a group of non-dairy vegetarians to discuss this diet and lifestyle. They needed a term for this type of eating, and 'dairyban,' 'vitan,' and 'benevore' were among the brainstormed words they rejected. They finally settled on the word 'vegan,' which contained the first three and last two letters of the word 'vegetarian.'

1950: The Cabbage Soup Diet

As the name implies, it's a diet allowing you only to eat cabbage soup. It is a short-term weight loss plan.

1952: Marilyn Monroe

Today, many women might go on juice cleanses or detox diets; Marilyn Monroe did differently. In a 1952 edition of Pageant Magazine, Marilyn highlighted her eating regimen in an article 'How I Stay in Shape.' Whether traveling or staying at home, she always started her day with a glass of two raw eggs mixed with warm milk.

1962: Weight Watchers

Still a massive organization today, Weight Watchers took flight in the 1960s, offering products and services to help people lose weight.

1963: The Atkins Diet

Dr. Robert Atkins created this diet, advising people to go on a low-carb, high-protein diet. The Atkins Diet is still followed by many today.

1966: The Sleeping Beauty Diet

The idea behind this diet is to sleep more throughout the day, not to be awake and to eat food. The more you sleep, the less food you consume, and the more weight you lose. It led some people to take a sleep aid, or even pills like Xanax, to help them fall asleep for longer.

1975: The Paleo Diet

A diet consisting of grass-fed meats, fruits, vegetables, and whole foods like nuts and seeds. The Paleo diet is still very popular today and I'll be reviewing it in more detail in a later chapter.

1980: Fruitarianism

As the name alludes to, it's a diet based solely on eating fruits and sometimes nuts. Around the birth of this diet, the Late Steve Jobs, founder of Apple, tried this way of eating.

The 1990s: Juice Fasting

The idea of cleansing your body through drinking only juices rose to fame around this time. Only drink fruit juices for a few days to 'cleanse your body.'

1992: The DASH Diet

The National Institute of Health in the USA funded research on this diet in conjunction with Harvard University. The Dietary Approaches to Stop Hypertension (DASH) diet is recommended to treat or prevent hypertension or high blood pressure. It is said to help reduce blood pressure by consuming a diet rich in vegetables, fruits, whole grains, and lean protein. In addition, the diet recommends reducing the consumption of red meat, salt, added sugars, and fat.

1993: The Pescatarian Diet

This diet centers around eating fish as your primary source of protein while foregoing chicken, beef, and dairy. Pescatarians may also eat vegetables, grains, and pulses.

1995: The Zone Diet

Once popular among many celebrities, the Zone Diet revolves around eating a balanced mix of proteins, carbs, and fats at every meal.

1996: The Blood Type Diet

Created by naturopath Peter D'Adamo, he believed the foods you eat react chemically with your blood type. It supposedly allows you to be healthier and lose weight more efficiently.

2000: The Dukan Diet

Another diet promoting low carbs, the Dukan Diet, emphasizes consuming more proteins and fats than anything else.

2002: The Alkaline Diet

Also known as the 'Alkaline Ash Diet,' it's a way of eating that allows for pH levels in the body (and acidity) to be altered, helping proponents of the diet improve their health and well-being.

2003: The South Beach Diet

Dr. Arthur Agatston, an American cardiologist, adopted some ideas from the Atkins Diet to develop his own – The South Beach Diet. Rather than keeping things low-carb, he advised eating low-glycemic index carbs and consuming lean proteins and unsaturated fats.

2012: Intermittent Fasting (16:8 Diet/5:2 Diet)

Intermittent fasting is all about eating within a certain period, or 'window of eating.' The 16:8 diet is structured to fast for 16 hours a day and consume all caloric needs in the remaining eight hours. The 5:2 diet is about eating what you want for five days, then restricting your calorie intake to 500 calories per day for two days.

So, now that you have an idea about the history of dieting and some of the most popular diets ever created, let me dive deeper into today's most popular diets.

"Eating is so intimate. It's very sensual. When you invite someone to sit at your table and you want to cook for them, you're inviting a person into your life."

—Maya Angelou

Chapter 2
Why Do We Eat?

Have you ever considered why you eat the way you do?

We often focus on what to eat, how much to eat, and even how to eat. But what about the why? *Why* do you eat?

We live in a world of plenty. Turn on Netflix and find an abundance of shows and movies. On the internet, we have access to endless information. As with most other things, there is also more than enough food.

We all eat for valid reasons, and it's more than just comfort or eating to satisfy our emotions.

If eating were as simple as turning on the TV to watch a show, we would not be living in a global obesity and diabetes epidemic.

So, what influences your food choices and decisions?

Let's start with the most obvious – hunger. This physiological need makes up one of the determinants of food choice. Your body needs energy and nutrients to survive, so it will always respond to your hunger levels.

We also eat because of taste. Think of a food you like to eat – do you eat it because of the nutrients it provides to your body, or because you enjoy the taste? Personally, while considering taste, I primarily eat foods because of the nutrition it provides to my body.

Our taste preferences are with us from the day we are born and develop over time. Everyone is different, and we all seem to have different tastes. It is the reason we all eat different foods. Our ethnicity partly influences it. For instance, those of Indian ethnicity prefer highly spiced foods while the more western ethnicities prefer milder flavors.

On a positive note, you can develop your taste buds to enjoy healthy foods. It just takes time and practice to eat healthily.

Do you have a childhood memory of a specific food that you loved? Fond memories of food also make us want to eat. Any emotional attachment to a particular food, or something we have eaten which gives us joy, will likely make us eat that food. There have been times where I've given in to eating a certain kind of chips or chocolate not because I'm craving them per se, but because they spark a childhood memory. What specific food did you love as a child? Have you eaten it recently because of its sentimental value?

Eating with our eyes undoubtedly influences our food choices. How many times have you eaten food just because it looks delicious? I am sure this has happened more times than you care to admit. Think about feeling full and satisfied after a great meal, but then the waiter pushed the dessert cart around. No matter how full you were, you probably gave in just because you saw the desserts on offer. We first eat with our eyes and then our mouth.

Cost and convenience also play a major part in our food decisions. After a long and stressful day, the last thing you want to think about is what to cook, so you'll order food instead. Maybe you're on a strict budget and opt for low-cost meals. Regardless, timesaving food choices play a part for anyone with limited time for grocery shopping and cooking.

Believe it or not, your personality can affect the way you eat. Are you the type of person who needs a list or meal plan highlighting the meals you should eat in a day? Or do you need flexibility in your daily diet? Understanding your personality type will help you better understand your food choices. As always, do what works best for you.

On that note, emotions play a massive part in our food choices. Emotional eating is common, and stress, boredom, sadness, and anger can trigger you to over or under-eat, depending on your personality.

Your mood influences your food choices and intake; your food choices and also have intake influence your mood. These influences are related to our attitude toward food. It's a constant struggle between eating certain foods and being conscious of your weight and calorie intake. People who diet or heavily restrict themselves feel guilty for not eating the foods they think they should be eating. This type of food restriction can also increase the desire for particular foods, otherwise known as food cravings.

Your attitude, beliefs, and knowledge affect the way you eat. Some people don't have the knowledge about what to eat. Others genuinely believe food won't harm them, so they'll eat whatever they want. On the flip side, you might already believe in the power of nutrition and the phrase 'you are what you eat' – so you make rational and healthy food decisions.

Last but certainly not least, your environment influences the way you eat. Typically, we eat more when we are around our family and friends and away from home. But this also depends on the type of people you surround yourself with; with more health-conscious friends or family, you'll tend to eat more nutritiously. If the opposite is true, you'll most likely give in to what they're eating. It is important to surround yourself with like-minded people who share similar goals. Positively managing your environment can increase the success rate throughout your health journey.

Your behavior toward food is a complex situation. Many factors drive what you eat and why you eat. To live a healthy lifestyle with more control and certainty, take a step back and analyze your decision-making process. A quick and easy way to do this is through food tracking. Use a food diary to log all the meals you eat on a given day and write down the trigger to what and why you ate. Knowing the drivers behind your food choices can identify traits to help you make healthy choices and eat better overall.

"The second day of a diet is always easier than the first. By the second day, you're off it."
—Jackie Gleason

Chapter 3
Why Do Diets Fail?

Dr. Marcio Griebeler, an endocrinologist affiliated with several hospitals in Ohio, including Cleveland Clinic, believes that your body is programmed to be at a certain weight, or 'weight set point.' He says, "Your body is fighting to maintain your weight as it was before dieting, and factors such as genes, hormones, behavior, and environment affect your weight set point."

"A fad diet won't change your set point. It's just restricting calories," Dr. Griebeler says. "Your body is very efficient. You can successfully lose weight for a while, but at some point, it simply adjusts to needing fewer calories to function."

When this happens, weight loss will stop and perhaps even increase unless you further restrict your calorie intake more than the diet recommends. Unfortunately, you won't be heading in the right direction if you go this way.

If you've invested in a diet plan, you're wasting your time and money.

Being overweight or obese, as per the body mass index, calls for action to alleviate symptoms of specific health issues. The body mass index (BMI) is a person's body weight in kilograms divided by the square of their height in meters. It is a measuring tool to screen people for weight categories that may be indicative of health issues.

By calculating your BMI using your weight and height, you'll understand which weight category you fall into:

<18.5 = **underweight**
18.5 – 24.5 = **normal weight**
25 – 29.9 = **overweight**
>30 = **obese**

Don't worry if you calculate your BMI and fall under the overweight or obese category. Unless you are actually overweight or obese, BMIs are typically an indication. For example, tall and muscular people may have a higher weight, ultimately leading to a higher BMI. Although they may not necessarily be overweight or obese, their BMI may be high because of their stature and muscle mass.

Back to the point, losing weight through a strict diet definitely helps the obese, diabetics and others suffering from medical issues. However, for clinically healthy individuals (those without medical conditions) looking to lose weight, lose fat, or simply live and feel healthy, there is no need for dieting.

What do you think about when you hear the word 'diet?' I'm sure you think of calorie restriction, starvation, removing foods you enjoy, removing foods from certain food groups, and the list goes on. But unfortunately, nothing associated with a diet is positive other than the potential of you losing weight for a short period. So why do it in the first place?

Let me quote another definition of a diet from the Cambridge English Dictionary. A diet is 'an eating plan in which someone eats less food, or only particular types of food because they want to become thinner or for medical reasons.'

Indeed, diets are a short-term solution. Those looking to prepare their summer body for the holidays, marriage, or a wedding, are the ones who would consider a diet. When Beyoncé tried the Lemonade Diet, she prepared herself for Coachella, a music festival in California. Indeed, diets are quick fixes and not a lifestyle. They're not designed to change your mindset around nutrition nor your eating habits and behaviors. Diets are designed for short-term rapid weight loss.

Most people have an all-or-nothing approach to diets – they'll go extreme for two weeks following the diet religiously, then guess what happens? They'll relapse, and the body will go back to its original state. Again, it's because diets are designed for you to go out of your way and follow a particular eating style, rather than focusing on small incremental changes that can last a lifetime. You can easily go on a diet and lose some weight, but if you don't change your habits, which is hard to do, you will regain all the weight you tried so hard to lose.

At the same time, we associate diets with 'less.' Consuming fewer calories, eating less chocolate, eating fewer carbs, eating less fat, you name it. The fact is that diets are meant for you to eat less, especially eating less of the foods you enjoy and eating less food within specific food groups (i.e., carbohydrates).

Eating less of a particular food or food group and holding yourself back from foods you enjoy will not only add to mental and physical stress, which I'll discuss in later chapters of the book; it makes things unsustainable. How long can you go without eating carbs? How long can you hold yourself back from chocolate, sweets, or foods you love? How long can you go with only drinking juices?

Coupling the idea of less with unsustainability leads to a lack of enjoyment – a third reason why diets don't work. Life is too short; we need to enjoy every moment and enjoy our food! There's nothing better than dining with family and friends, and enjoying eating at a restaurant and the vibe it brings. What about a lazy Saturday or Sunday, ordering Chinese take-out and eating noodles straight from the box? There's nothing like it.

By going on diets, rest assured you'll feel restricted. Go back and review the diets I mentioned in chapter 1 and consider the many limitations they bring. For example, one diet recommends you only drink juices; the other tells you only to eat fruits. One recommends you eat low-carbs, but another tells you to eat carbs and only eat low-glycemic index carbs. Oh, and how about you follow a diet where you can only drink cabbage soup. Really?

Restrictions, quick fixes, unsustainability and a lack of enjoyment – these are the reasons why diets never work. They fall short as a sustainable lifestyle choice to lose weight and maintain overall health and wellbeing. You may lose weight in the short term, but that's as far as it goes. I assure you; the weight will come back to haunt you.

"I've been through my highs, I've been through my lows; I've been through the gamut of all things in this business. Being too thin. Being bigger. I've been criticized for being on both sides of the scale. It's noise I block out automatically. I love my body."

—Christina Aguilera

Chapter 4
The Deprived Body

As Dr. Lulu Hunt, the queen of calories puts it – weight loss is nothing more than an energy (or calorie) balance. Here's what you need to know about the relationship between calories and your weight.

To maintain your weight, you need to be consuming the same amount of calories as you are burning. To lose weight, you need to put your body in a calorie deficit by burning more calories than you consume. Weight gain results from a calorie surplus, consuming more calories than you burn. These are the basic principles behind weight management.

You can eat five meals a day, maintain a daily calorie deficit, and still lose weight. There's absolutely no need to be juice cleansing, fasting, or consuming a minimum prescribed number of calories per day.

What is a recommended calorie deficit? A calorie deficit of 500 to 1000 is needed to lose weight healthily. The magnitude of your deficit is dependent on your weight loss goal. Typically, a deficit of 500 calories per day is the general recommendation. For example, to lose one pound of fat, you need a 3,500-calorie deficit per week – that's 500 calories per day. Those who are obese need to increase their daily deficit slightly.

I would never recommend a deficit of greater than 1,000 calories. Many people starting their weight loss journey believe that skipping meals to lower their calorie intake means they'll lose weight faster. However, what they don't know is that too big of a calorie deficit may backfire. Every single function in the human body requires energy (calories); this includes regulating body temperature, breathing, heart rate, movement, digestion, and more.

You even burn calories at rest. Resting Metabolic Rate (RMR) is often used interchangeably with Basal Metabolic Rate (BMR). As the name suggests, PMR is the rate at which your body burns energy at complete rest, and your BMR is the minimum number of calories your body burns simply to survive.

There are many equations used to calculate RMR, though these equations are rough estimates. To truly understand how many calories you burn at rest requires a method known as indirect calorimetry. This technique helps you understand the amount of heat produced by the body by measuring oxygen consumption and carbon dioxide production. It's a non-invasive and very accurate way of measuring your RMR.

I like to use the Mifflin St. Jeor equation in my practice, as it's the most accurate equation for measuring RMR. Here are the equations for men and women:

Men

RMR (kcal/day) = (10 * weight in kg) + (6.25 * height in cm) − (5 * age in years) + 5 (kcal/day)

Women

RMR (kcal/day) = (10 * weight in kg) + (6.25 * height in cm) − (5 * age in years) − 161 (kcal/day)

RMR helps your body perform the most basic functions while at rest. The functions like breathing, circulating blood, and basic cognitive functions all require energy. Everyone has a different RMR, depending on your weight, height, age, gender, and body composition, as per the equation. Typically, taller, heavier, and more muscular individuals will have a higher RMR as they need more energy to maintain their bodies at rest than smaller and thinner individuals.

Take a minute and calculate your RMR.

Hence, your RMR is the minimum amount of calories the body needs to function at rest. So why does an excessive calorie deficit hinder the body? To demonstrate this point, I'm going to use my metrics. When writing this book, I'm 32 years of age, with a weight of 68kg and a height of 165cm. Here's my RMR:

RMR (kcal/day) = (10 * 65) + (6.25 * 165) − (5 * 32) + 5 = 1,556cal/day

It is the rate at which my body utilizes energy to perform the simplest functions. With dieting and extreme calorie cuts, numerous people will consume less than their body needs to function at rest. So if I'm burning 1,556 calories at rest and only consuming 1,000 calories, my body may respond by saying, 'okay, why am I working so hard when I'm not getting the necessary energy I need to perform at the most basic level?' What happens then? Your body's metabolism starts to slow down.

Metabolism is how your body converts food into energy to perform both simple and complex body functions. All the food we eat contains nutrients that our body transfers into units of heat or calories. The calories (or energy) we receive from the breakdown of food are used immediately to perform functions in the body or stored for later use (usually as fat).

In fact, the phenomenon of a slower metabolism during a weight loss journey is explained by a term called adaptive thermogenesis (AT). Your body burns calories to maintain its weight. Even the maintenance of fat storage in the body requires energy. The heavier you are, the more calories your body needs. When you lose weight, your body burns fewer calories, which is a normal response. In certain instances, though, a decrease in calorie burn can be explained through more than just a loss in body weight. Adaptive thermogenesis can cause a slower resting metabolic rate by reducing the body's heat production to save energy and keep you from starving when calories are heavily restricted.

There are a few things that can affect your metabolism:

Genetics: some people are born with genes that allow them to have a faster metabolism than others.

Gender: men have a higher RMR than women. Typically, men have a higher muscle mass and lower body fat mass, which increases their metabolism.

Age: as we age, our metabolism decreases. Metabolism typically starts to slow down in our 20s.

Weight: the more you weigh, the higher your metabolism.

Height: taller people have a greater body surface area than shorter people.

Body fat percentage: those with a higher body fat percentage have a lower metabolism.

Diet: Diets promoting a high calorie deficit can decrease metabolism by around 20–30%. Another point to help you realize why diets are harmful.

Exercise: an increase in exercise increases metabolism, and lower activity levels lower metabolism.

Body temperature: Every increase of 0.5 degrees Celsius raises metabolism by around 7%. The higher the body's core temperature, the greater the body has to work to regulate all body functions.

External temperature: very cold temperatures can increase the body's metabolism. An extended period in the heat can have the same effect.

Thyroid Glands: thyroxine is a hormone produced by the thyroid glands. The more thyroxine produced, the greater the body's metabolism. The less thyroxine produced, the lower the metabolism.

If your metabolism slows down, then clearly, you're not allowing your body to perform at its best. All metabolic processes require calories to build tissue (anabolism) and break down tissue and food substrates for energy (catabolism). So what is the consequence of a slower metabolism? Catabolism, which weakens your immune system, bone health, muscle health, digestive health, and nervous system. You may also experience rapid hair loss, poor skin health, weak nails, and feel lethargic.

I've only explained the negative relationship between diet and physical health purely from the angle of RMR. There's also a term known as Total Energy Expenditure (TEE), the total amount of calories you burn in a day. TEE is the sum of your RMR, thermogenic effect of food (TEF), non-exercise activity thermogenesis (NEAT), exercise post-energy consumption (EPOC), and finally exercise (E). The equation is:

TEE = RMR + TEF + NEAT + EPOC + E

To make things more straightforward, the thermic effect of food is the calories your body burns to digest, absorb, and metabolize the food you eat. Non-exercise activity thermogenesis is the calories burned for daily activities other than sleep, eating, or exercise. For example, activities like house chores, walking from the car to the office, and getting up to grab the TV remote, are all considered NEAT.

For EPOC, I like to use the analogy of a car and its engine. After driving for a long period, once you turn the engine off, it remains hot and slowly cools to its normal temperature. This is EPOC but in relation to exercise and calories. Once you complete a workout, especially at a high intensity, your body will continue to burn calories until it reaches its resting state. Simply put, it's the amount of oxygen required to bring your body back to its normal restorative state or homeostasis.

Exercise is the last factor included in TEE. An activity multiplier is a varying level of multipliers which represent the amount of activity you do in one week:

Sedentary = 1.2 (little or no exercise, desk job)

Lightly active = 1.375 (light exercise/sports 1–3 days/week)

Moderately active = 1.55 (moderate exercise/sports 6–7 days/week)

Very active = 1.725 (hard exercise every day, or exercising twice a day)

Extra active = 1.9 (hard exercise two or more times per day, or training for a marathon, or triathlon, etc.)

To measure your TEE, take your RMR and multiply it by the activity multiplier to get the number of calories you burn in a day given your exercise, as shown below:

Sedentary = RMR x 1.2 (little or no exercise, desk job)

Lightly active = RMR x 1.375 (light exercise/sports 1–3 days/week)

Moderately active = RMR 1.55 (moderate exercise/sports 6–7 days/week)

Very active = RMR x 1.725 (hard exercise every day, or exercising twice a day)

Extra active = RMR 1.9 (hard exercise two or more times per day, or training for marathon, or triathlon, etc.)

Go ahead and calculate your TEE.

Since I burn 1,556 calories at rest, the amount of calories burned per day is 2,411 calories (I multiplied my RMR by 1.55 as I train six times per week). So, continuing my example, given that I burn 2,411 calories and consume 1,000 calories, I'm essentially putting my body in a deficit of 1,411 That's a big deficit!

Aside from the consequences of your metabolism slowing down, your body begins to produce and store fat under a big calorie deficit. Fat is the body's way to protect and provide insulation for our organs; if your body is not getting sufficient calories to function, it will produce fat to protect your organs and keep you surviving when food is limited. In fact, this is due to AT once again. From a survival point of view, a slower metabolism due to AT makes sense, but from a weight loss standpoint, it could be an issue. Adaptive thermogenesis can play a big role in the high rates of weight regain following dieting.

Dr. Griebeler said, "Research tells us that yo-yo dieting can negatively affect your metabolism. It doesn't matter the diet: low-carb, low-fat, ketogenic, whatever. We see rebound weight gain almost every time."

If you think that skipping meals and lowering calorie intake will help you lose weight and fat, think again. You may lose weight in the first couple of weeks, but over time, you'll hit a plateau before gaining weight and fat while facing other potential health issues – another reason why diets backfire.

What's more? By burning calories while restricting your body from what it needs to perform, you will experience a decrease in exercise performance, and as a result, recovery will also be impaired. I'm sure you've heard many times that it's not what you do in the gym that will provide you with the training benefits; it's what you do outside of the gym which will ultimately have the biggest impact on your performance, recovery, and what we call 'gains.' Again, suppose you're lowering your calorie intake drastically. In that case, you're not providing your body with the calories and nutrients it needs for *repairing* damaged muscle fibers, *refueling* the muscle with energy, and even *rehydration* – the 3 Rs required for recovery.

Extreme calorie cuts won't provide sufficient protein (and calories) to build and repair muscle. To provide you with energy during extreme calorie restriction, your body will begin to dig into glycogen, the stored form of carbohydrates in the muscle and liver for energy. Once your glycogen stores are depleted, you will lose water, as every one gram of carbohydrate you consume is attached to three grams of water.

Depending on the diet you follow, extreme calorie cuts can also impair blood sugar levels in the body. For example, let's say you do a juice cleanse – the rapid and regular sugar surges from the juices can cause spikes and drops of sugar in the blood. Over time, this can lead to insulin resistance, which can, in turn, lead to type 2 diabetes.

You may be dieting and doing really well, losing weight and feeling good. Eventually and inevitably, you start seeing no change in your weight and may even see an increase. You and your diet are like the ultimate catch-22.

"Look, I eat really well, and I work out, but I also indulge when I want to. I don't starve myself in an extremist way. You're not taking away my coffee or my dairy or my glass of wine because I'd be devastated."
—Jennifer Aniston

Chapter 5
The Starved Brain

Can the type of food you eat affect your mental health? Absolutely.

Does the amount of food you eat affect your mental health? Absolutely.

The brain is the body's most complex organ. It is made up of millions of cells, known as neurons, which react together with the help of chemicals called neurotransmitters to shape our thoughts, feelings, and attitude.[2] Neurotransmitters are the body's chemical messengers, which work together to improve cognitive function, from focus and concentration to managing our breathing and heart rate. The performance of neurotransmitters is dependent on nutrition. The better the quality of nutrition, the more powerfully and efficiently the neurotransmitters work. Therefore, giving the brain the right food and the right nutrients is essential to our existence. To experience optimal mental health and maximize our brain's potential, you need to be focusing on eating well and eating enough.

The previous chapter described the relationship between diets and physical health, highlighting how diets negatively impact your physical health. Indeed, poor physical health has been shown to lead to poor mental health and wellbeing. [50] For example, poor nutrition can lead to health problems such as obesity. A 2010 systematic review on the relationship between obesity and depression found a two-way association; those who were obese had a 55% increased risk of developing depression, whereas those who were depressed had a 58% increased risk of becoming obese. [42]

Fad diets prescribe either too little food or exclude certain food groups; it leads to food deprivation which tips the body into semi-starvation, leading to physical deprivation. This deprivation has a profound effect on moods and overall function. When deprived or starved of food, the body begins to slow down its metabolic rate. The brain operates at a high metabolic rate, requiring a large amount of nutrients and energy. The brain is improperly fueled by food deprivation and starvation from dieting, affecting transmission, and function, making it weak and vulnerable. [53]

Many well-conducted studies worldwide have highlighted the relationship between diets and mental health disorders, such as depression and anxiety. We now know the importance of diet not only on physical health but also on mental health. A body of evidence shows that an unhealthy diet is indeed a risk factor for depression and anxiety.

As I talk about the relationship between diets and mental health, there is nothing more compelling than one of the most famous studies on diets and the brain, known as The Minnesota Starvation Experiment, conducted by Dr. Ancel Keys during World War II. Dr. Keys wanted to understand the 'biology of human starvation.'[33] Thirty-six young men agreed to participate in a year-long study after being exempt from armed service for ethical reasons. They took the young men into three stages: three months of preparation, six months of semi-starvation, and three months of refeeding. The young men were quite motivated as they wanted to help their companions fighting overseas deal with starvation. The purpose of the study was to learn how people would cope under semi-starvation conditions and how to refeed starving populations successfully.

Here's the first line of the study: "On November 19, 1944, 36 healthy young men entered the brick confines of the Laboratory of Physiological Hygiene at the University of Minnesota, where they were to embark on a grueling medical experiment." The brochure of the study read 'Will You Starve That They Be Better Fed?' [33]

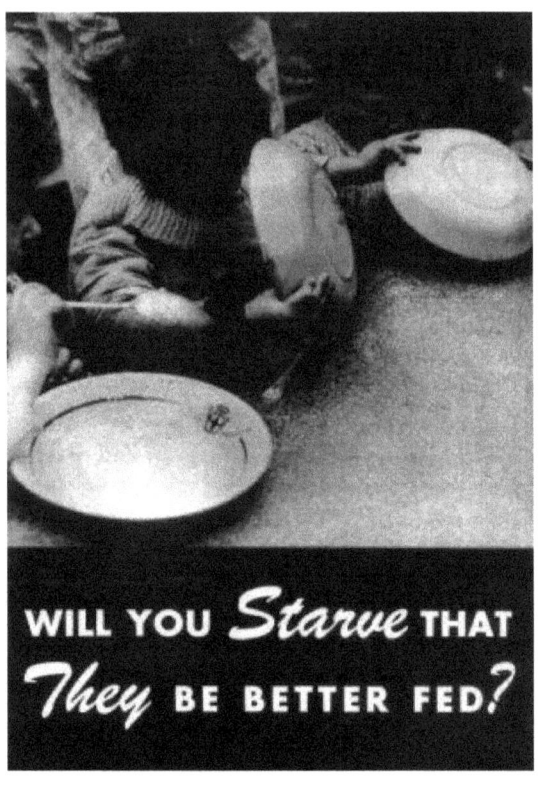

The young men lived in the dormitory at the University of Minnesota. Walking 22 miles each week was the exercise coupled with their restricted diets. Once the starvation period began, all food was prepared in the dorm, and the aim was to allow a weight loss of 25% of the subjects' bodyweight – around 1.1kg per week. For the first three months, subjects consumed 3,200 calories per day and then reduced their intake to 1,600 calories per day during the semi-starvation period. Their nutrition plan consisted of foods such as root vegetables, potatoes, bread, and macaroni.

Unsurprisingly, the young men went through horrible experiences. They felt lethargic, irritable, and anxious, especially after seeing their eating schedule for the following week. One participant, Daniel Peacock, remembered what it was like in the cafeteria line after seeing the person in front of him getting more food:

"We were given our food along a cafeteria line, and if the guy ahead of you is given five slices of bread, that's pretty hard to conceal. And if you're only getting three, that's pretty touchy." He also spoke of the anxiety that accompanied the Friday night posting of the upcoming week's rations. "Every Friday late in the day…they would post a list of all our names and what our rations would be for the following week…[the] calories…either minus or plus…Some of us…we'd go off to a movie. In other words, we delayed seeing that list; we dreaded seeing that list for fear that it was certainly going to reduce our rations…It's pretty darn certain that it's going to be bad news because we're supposed to be descending."

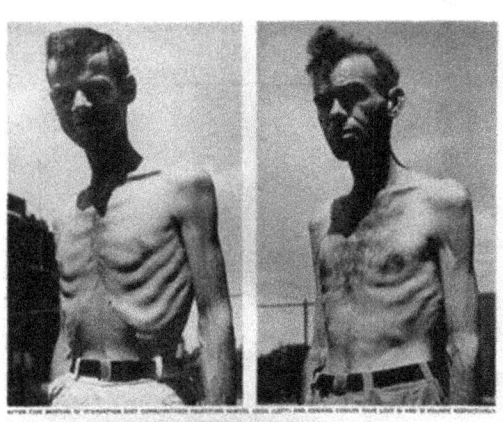

After being 'unable to take any more,' one subject excused himself from the study. Due to this, they implemented a buddy system whereby no one could leave the dormitory unaccompanied. One subject, Jasper Garner, was thankful because he was getting weaker by the day. "Before the buddy system, I was in Dayton's department store downtown going to go in. It's got a rotating door. I couldn't push it. I got stuck. I had to wait until somebody came along. And then the other one was, you know, the library doors. Oh, you know, they're big, and I couldn't pull them. I had to wait until somebody...let me scoot in after."

Another participant, Carlyle Fredrick, said, "Noticing what's wrong with everybody else, even your best friend. Their idiosyncrasies became great big deals...little things that wouldn't bother me before or after would really make me upset."

Marshall Sutton noted, "We were impatient waiting in line if we had to...and we'd get disturbed with each other's eating habits at times...I remember going to a friend at night and apologizing and saying, 'Oh, I was terrible today, and you know, let's go to sleep with other thoughts in our minds.' We became, in a sense, more introverted, and we had less energy. I knew where all the elevators were in the buildings."

Aside from facing physical issues like muscle soreness, hair loss and dizziness, the subjects couldn't concentrate and had to withdraw from university classes. They became obsessed with food, creating food rituals (which those with eating disorders do, by the way) and even adding water to their plate to make their food last longer. Robert Willoughby remembered the ridiculous things they used to do. "Eating became a ritual...Some people diluted their food with water to make it seem like more. Others would put each little bite and hold it in their mouth a long time to savor it. So eating took a long time."

They collected cookbooks and recipes to visually indulge in food, mainly Carlyle Fredrick, who had collected 100 books by the end of the study. He said, "I don't know many other things in my life that I looked forward to being over with any more than this experiment. And it wasn't so much...because of the physical discomfort, but because it made food the most important thing in one's life...food became the one central and only thing really in one's life. And life is pretty dull if that's the only thing. I mean, if you went to a movie, you weren't particularly interested in the love scenes, but you noticed every time they ate and what they ate."

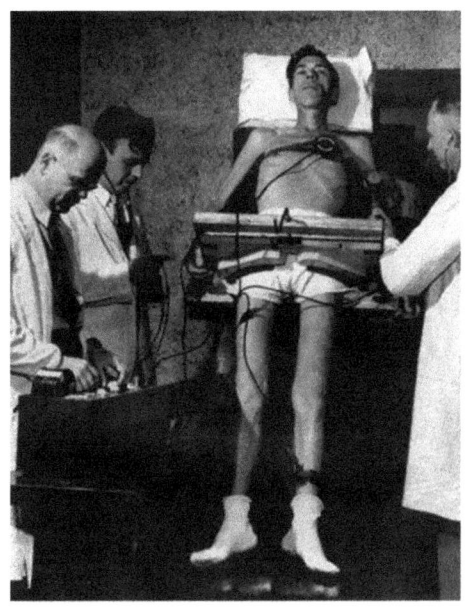

One of the subjects bought doughnuts and handed them out to children in the street just to watch them eat. The Minneapolis Star-Journal noted, "One of the men was walking past a bakery and was so tempted by the rich odors wafting from the place that he rushed in and bought a dozen doughnuts. He gave them to children in the street and watched with relish as they ate them."

The study initially permitted chewing gum, but when the subjects began to chew 40 pieces a day, the study's authors decided to stop this to prevent any manipulation of the study results.

Only 32 of the original 36 subjects completed the study. One excused himself from the study, and another broke the rules, scrapping for food in garbage cans and eating sundaes at shops. Two men were admitted into a psychiatric hospital—one committed suicide, and the other cut off three of his fingers.

During the three-month refeeding period, the symptoms of lethargy and dizziness improved, but they continued to experience hunger and weakness. Jasper Garner described it as a 'year-long cavity.' After being released from the study, one subject was hospitalized to get his stomach pumped following binge eating. Roscoe Hinkle put on substantial weight even though he experienced weight loss during the study. He said, "Boy did I add weight. Well, that was flab. You don't have muscle yet. And get[ting] the muscle back again, boy, that's no fun."

The Minnesota Starvation Experiment compiles a lot of stories into one. It reminds us of the privilege we have of having access to food easily and readily. It reminds us that we can eat food if we are hungry. Hunger, through dieting, is harsh and ultimately leads to a plethora of negative consequences.

I'm sure you can already pinpoint some important takeaways from this study. First and foremost, diets can make you go insane, especially if you put your body under semi or extreme starvation through heavily restricting calories. From a focus perspective, heavily restricting calories impairs your ability to concentrate, hindering your reaction time, decision-making skills, and problem-solving abilities.

Your food intake affects your mood. Feeling irritable, moody, anxious, stressed, and unhappy are among the many emotions you may experience. In addition, you may experience a lack of enthusiasm, motivation, and alertness. Interestingly, the calorie restriction may also affect your attitude and behavior. Like the Minnesota Starvation Experiment participants, constantly thinking about food, creating unusual food rituals, and an eternal feeling of hunger are among other symptoms experienced.

Furthermore, you can either develop eating disorders or adopt the habits of those who suffer from eating disorders. According to the National Eating Disorders Collection, "dieting is one of the most common forms of disordered eating." I mentioned previously the notion of significantly cutting back on calories leading to a slower metabolism. A reduction in the body's metabolic rate can lead to binge and overeating behaviors, resulting in weight gain and obesity. On the flip side, going under extreme calorie cuts may also lead to disorders such as anorexia nervosa, characterized by undereating and fear of weight gain, and bulimia nervosa, characterized by binge eating followed by purging (vomiting).

Furthermore, food deprivation can enhance expressions of mental health symptoms. The Dutch Hunger Winter Famine from October 1944 to May 1945 highlighted the importance of good nutrition during pregnancy.[60] The study looked at the effects of this famine on the offspring of pregnant women during this period. The study authors looked at the relationship between this famine and the risk of developing schizophrenia during the first trimester of pregnancy. Between 1978 and 1989, they found a two-fold increase between men and women exposed to the prenatal famine as opposed to those who weren't.

Emotional Health

Whether you like it or not, dieting impacts your emotional health and, ultimately, your social life. Everything is connected; the mental, the physical and the emotional. By negatively impacting the mental and physical, it will skew the emotional.

As I mentioned in the previous chapter, the brain has a high metabolic rate – it's always turned on, controlling all aspects of your mind, body and soul. The brain's fuel comes from food, and the fuel quality depends on the food quality. The quality of foods you eat directly correlates to the structure and function of your brain, and ultimately your emotions.

Have you felt *hangry (hungry and angry)* before? I'm sure you have. It's a clear example of how food can play a role in emotions. Go too long without eating, and your blood sugar level drops, inviting feelings of anger, frustration, and light-headedness. Then once you've finally eaten, you feel happy again. That's because food can help produce serotonin, the feel-good hormone which makes us feel happy and calm.

The gut produces 90% of our serotonin.[19] The Enteric Nervous System links the brain and gut, showing us a clear link between the two. By dieting and restricting foods, be it a food group or specific food, you deprive your gut of the essential nutrients it needs to feel nourished and energized.

The gastrointestinal tract is lined with a hundred million neurons, which all work together to help digestion of foods and help guide emotions. There are billions of good bacteria in the gut microbiome that influence these neurons' function, impacting many aspects of our health. Gut neurons also help protect and strengthen the intestinal wall lining, helping fight off any toxins and bad bacteria in the gut. In doing so, the gut can enhance nutrients' absorption, activating the neural pathways between the gut and the brain. This process, of course, helps with improving our mood.

Think of the last time you were dieting. How did you feel? How was your social life? How many invitations did you turn down because you did not have your act together and feared the emotional struggles that may follow? Have you ever found that the eating limitations your diet prescribes have made you feel alone in social environments by forcing you to eat differently than everyone else?

When dieting, the restrictions and limitations placed on you lead to personal emotional battles; some dieters may isolate themselves to avoid food temptations. This behavior can lead to low self-esteem, which brings many other complications, all caused by restrictive dieting. For example, being more critical of others, reduced care to create social relationships, a loss of sense of humor, and feelings of social inadequacy.

What happens if you don't see results when dieting? What emotional trauma follows? Believe it or not, but some people end up hating themselves because of the lack of results. First, they'll feel confused and frustrated because they expect to lose weight by barely eating, but then don't. Then, they'll develop an overwhelming feeling of failure for not achieving their goals. People often look at themselves in the mirror and feel ashamed, leading them to stay at home, avoiding any social events. If it's summertime, they won't want to go to the beach and expose their body. I know there may be other underlying psychological issues causing this, but it mainly originates from dieting.

If someone you know seems more stressed than usual, it could very well mean they are dieting. Dieting just adds so much additional stress to your life. The constant worry about what you can (and can't) eat, the daily weigh-ins, calorie counting, the fear of gaining weight, the obsession with losing weight – all cause stress in the body. Today we are faced with the worry of social media. We live in a world of plenty, and there are plenty of models and influencers on Instagram who mess with your mind because of your deep desire to look like them. The idea of not being as 'fit as him' or as 'thin as her' adds even more stress. What happens in our body once stress occurs? Cortisol levels increase. Some cortisol is good for the body, but too much cortisol can lead to weight gain. It's a cycle. Similar to how sleep deprivation can affect our day and make it more stressful, a diet causing food deprivation, and hunger can affect our emotional stability.

Diets do not consider every individual's requirements, including their lifestyle, food preferences, or exercise levels. Because of this, dieting leads to feelings of constant hunger, mood swings, low energy, and overall poor and emotional mental health. It also leads to hating yourself and hating life. The idea of having so many restrictions and limitations will paint a negative outlook, and you simply won't enjoy life; you'll miss out on fun moments with your family and friends, and you'll miss out on eating good food. After all, we need to eat to satisfy our hunger, we need to eat for pleasure, and we need to eat to provide our body with the nutrients it needs to stay strong and healthy. Above all, we need to enjoy the simple pleasures of life like food.

"The very fact that we are having a national conversation about what we should eat, that we are struggling with the question about what the best diet is, is symptomatic of how far we have strayed from the natural conditions that gave rise to our species, from the simple act of eating real, whole, fresh food."

—Mark Hyman

Chapter 6
The Dangers of Supplements

What if you can take a pill and burn fat? Would you drink only teas to detox and cleanse your body? How about mixing a powdery drink for more muscle and less fat?

While many diets sound sexy with the unbelievable transformations they promise and the profound results you'll experience, you need to think twice about these options. Don't be fooled by the marketing stunts, because after all, dieting can be quite dangerous, especially if undertaken without any guidance.

It's easy to get tempted from reading things online or when an influencer promotes a supplement or a specific way of eating. Instead, you need to do your due diligence and research the diets you contemplate following, making sure they're safe, but also to ensure you follow them correctly without harming yourself.

It's clear to you now that dieting can be pretty dangerous—harming your mental, physical and emotional health. What about the diets that promote products and supplements in parallel to restricted eating regimens?

The motivation behind the supplement industry is money. The industry skyrocketed from a $20 billion industry in 2004 into a $130 billion industry today. This number is expected to continue rising.

In the US, herbal, sports (i.e., protein powders), and micronutrient supplements are all considered under the Dietary Supplement Health and Education Act of 1994. Pills, powders and supplements which claim to boost weight loss, detox the body and help you burn fat have little government oversight over their safety and efficacy. The Food and Drug Administration (FDA) can oversee dietary supplements, having manufacturers remove their products from the market if they are deemed unsafe. However, after new legislation came into effect on October 15, 1995, any dietary supplements introduced into the market do not have to be tested for their safety or approved by the FDA.[20] Thus, while supplements have to mention the ingredients on the nutrition label, we don't know whether or not the supplement is safe to use, whether the mentioned ingredients actually exist, or whether additional ingredients are added. Simply put, the supplement industry is not regulated.

Taking supplements can be dangerous, especially in conjunction with a restrictive diet. You don't always know the supplement's exact ingredients, and if you are unaware of the correct dosage, you may very well be on your way to the emergency room. A study published in the New England Journal of Medicine examined the adverse effects of taking dietary supplements and their relation to the number of emergency room visits in the United States. They analyzed data for the ten years between January 1, 2004, and December 31, 2013, from 63 hospitals participating in the National Electronic Injury Surveillance System – Cooperative Adverse Drug Event Surveillance (NEISS-CADES) project led by the

Centers for Disease Control and Prevention (CDC), the FDA, and the Consumer Product Safety Commission.

The study's authors found the harmful effects of supplements responsible for an average of around 23,000 emergency room visits per year between 2004 and 2013. From these visits, 2,154 cases annually led to hospitalization. The supplement products most commonly used were multivitamins (33.6%), iron (11.8%), weight-loss supplements (10.4%), and supplements for sleep, sedation, and anxiolysis (8.8%). Of the emergency room visits caused by the implications of weight-loss products, 3,399 were female – almost three times that of male patients (1,223 emergency room visits). Regarding supplement-related adverse events, implications of weight-loss products were 30.4% among female patients, compared to 17.6% among male patients. On the other hand, the implications of bodybuilding products among male patients were 14.1%. More than half of these emergency room visits were among patients between the ages of five to 19 years of age (51.2%) and 20 to 34 years of age (56.4%).[20]

The most common symptoms caused by these products included cardiac symptoms associated with weight-loss products (42.9% of patients) and energy products (46% of patients). Implications for weight-loss and energy products that led to emergency room visits related to cardiac symptoms like palpitations, chest pain, or tachycardia was 71.8%. Most patients who visited the emergency room because of these symptoms were aged between 20 to 34 (58%).[20]

Suppose you replace food with supplements or undertake a restrictive diet. In that case, you may put your body in a state of malnourishment, meaning you will miss out on many nutrients which your body needs for optimal health and body growth and development.

What is the safe approach before considering using dietary supplements? Education. To be a healthier version of yourself requires a lot of self-care, and part of self-care is to be knowledgeable and aware of any supplement – even if it is herbal or natural.

First, always ask a pharmacist, doctor, or dietitian to review the supplement to ensure there are no harmful effects, either alone or in combination with other supplements or medication you're taking. Never take supplements without professional advice!

Second, make an effort to read the label. Check the ingredients and if there are any safety labels on the packaging. It is the only way to make an informed decision about what you're taking and how safe it is to use.

Third, you need to do a bit of research. Regardless of whether or not you get advice from a health professional, it's still good to do some reading yourself – it's part of the educational process.

When it comes to the safe use of supplements, it's essential to look out for company logos of those that batch-test supplements to ensure they are free from any harmful or illegal ingredients. Additionally, it is vital if you are a competitive athlete or a recreational athlete looking to stay drug-free.

There are three main global sports supplement-testing programs that ensure quality assurance before any supplement is released into the market – Informed Sport, Informed Choice, and the NSF.

These programs offer resources and services for you to understand how to search for supplements and know whether they are batch-tested. For example, you can go to the Informed Sport website and search for the supplement using the product or brand name or the batch number located on the packaging.

If the supplement appears on the website, you can be 99% sure that the supplement is safe to use and free of any harmful or illegal ingredients. In addition, if you see the label of one of these supplement testing programs on the packaging itself, you know the product or supplement has been batch tested.

If the supplement does not appear online, then I'd advise you not to consider taking it.

Self-care is not only about education; it's about eating the right types of food. If you eat a balanced, varied diet with healthy fats, lean proteins, good carbs, and colorful fruits and vegetables, you won't need to use any supplements.

In fact, only four groups of people qualify for the use of supplements: 1) anyone deficient in a particular vitamin or mineral, 2) pregnant women, 4) those who have a medical issue, 3) and the elderly, typically those above 70 years of age.

Another study led by researchers from the Harvard T.H Chan School of Public Health and Boston Children's hospital also showed intriguing results. The study authors analyzed data collected from 10,058 women and girls aged between 14 to 36 who participated in the Growing Up Study based in the US between the years of 2001 to 2016. They found that young women without eating disorders who took pills and laxatives for weight loss were more likely to be diagnosed with an eating disorder within 1–3 years in comparison with those who did not take any diet pills or laxatives.[41]

It's evident that using over-the-counter supplements, dietary pills and laxatives can cause serious health issues, including high blood pressure, liver, and kidney damage. The unregulated use of supplements may transition into eating disorders and dysregulated normal digestive function. It can also increase dependence on dietary pills and supplements to cope with dieting and weight loss.[41]

With all this being said, the dangers of using dietary supplements are vast. As you'll come to find out, many diets are fad diets, especially those which promote pills, teas, or any supplementary products. It's vital to do your due diligence and ensure you precisely understand what you are putting into your body. Take a step backward; it's important to realize that you can still lose weight and feel good without using and relying on supplements. Think about food before considering supplements. By eating food, you're not only getting energy; you're getting in so many nutrients that will boost your overall health and well-being. Supplements don't do that.

When it comes to nutrition, think of a cake. The base of the cake (the majority) is the foundation of nutrition. The foundation of nutrition is to eat clean, whole, and unprocessed foods the majority of the time. The cake's icing is adding in exercise and matching it with your nutrition – the two go hand in hand. Finally, the last thing you put on a cake is the sprinkles. Supplements are the last thing to think about when it comes to your nutrition. If you follow a sound nutrition regimen and don't diet, you won't need any supplements.

How many people do you know that start from the top of the cake or use supplements before thinking of improving their food choices and decisions? Some food for thought.

Section 2
A Review of Popular Diets on Weight-Loss

"It's one thing to lose weight, but it's another thing to eat healthily."

—Jennifer Hudson

Chapter 7
The Ketogenic Diet

Did you know that the ketogenic diet was the most Googled diet in 2018?

I wouldn't categorize the ketogenic (keto) diet as a *fad* diet because it's been used since the 1920s for medical reasons.

Many social media influencers promote the ketogenic diet without knowing the evidence behind it. They don't know what they're talking about most of the time; they're merely riding the keto wave to appear trendy and perhaps sell you products you don't need.

Is the ketogenic diet safe? Does it help with weight loss? Are there any side effects?

The basis of the ketogenic diet is high-fat and low-carb. The diet suggests consuming 70–80% of calories from fat, 10–20% from protein, and 5–10% from carbohydrates. Some studies suggest consuming less than 50 grams of carbohydrates per day, while others suggest consuming less than 20 grams per day.

The ketogenic diet essentially bans carbohydrates. Bread, potato, cereal, whole grains, legumes, and most fruits and vegetables are heavily restricted. If you eat one piece of bread, you've pretty much ruined the diet. Fruits like berries are the best types to consume (and in small portions only) as they are lower in sugar than other fruits. At the same time, the diet permits vegetables like leafy greens (kale, chard, spinach), broccoli, garlic, asparagus, cauliflower, Brussels sprouts[tc1], bell peppers, onion, mushrooms, cucumber and celery, but in limited quantities. However, they include a variety of saturated fats like butter, various cheeses, oil, bacon, fatty cuts of meat, and deli meats (which are highly processed). It also allows unsaturated (healthy) fats, including nuts, seeds, avocado, plant oils, and oily fish (i.e., salmon).

To understand the keto diet, you must understand how your body uses energy. The body's preferred energy source is carbohydrates, as they are easy to digest and provide a quick supply of energy. Once ingested, your body converts carbohydrates into glucose (sugar) which your brain uses for energy. The stored form of glucose, known as glycogen, is stored mainly in muscles and the liver. Muscle glycogen provides you with energy during exercise. Fat is a secondary energy source because it takes longer to digest and convert into energy. Lastly, our body also uses amino acids for energy. However, it only contributes 5% of our energy and is used mainly when the body is starved.

The brain needs a constant supply of glucose because it can't store glucose – it needs 120 grams daily, to be precise. When fasting or following the keto diet, the body begins to experience glucose depletion, and with time, glycogen is also depleted. The lack of glucose in the bloodstream causes insulin production to decrease, forcing the body to break down fat into molecules for energy. The liver then starts to produce ketones, becoming the primary fuel source for the brain and body.[50] This process is called ketosis, hence the name ketogenic diet.

There are some benefits to a keto diet, especially helping treat certain medical conditions. However, I want to discuss it purely from a *weight-loss* and lifestyle perspective targeted toward clinically healthy individuals. Most healthy people follow a keto diet because they heard it helps with weight loss, or maybe their friend lost weight on this plan, or a social media influencer promoted it, so they wanted to try it out themselves. But unfortunately, they don't have any idea of the science behind it.

Can you go without eating fruits and vegetables for a long time? I doubt it. Better yet, why on earth would you want to avoid eating these foods? With a vast reduction of these food groups, nutrient deficiencies may occur. For example, a lack of fruits, vegetables, and grains can lead to micronutrient deficiencies, mainly vitamin C, selenium, magnesium, and phosphorus. These foods also contain fiber, the lack of which may lead to constipation. They have so much nutritional value and provide numerous benefits to your body that it makes absolutely no sense to limit or exclude these foods from your diet.

Also, consuming 75% of your calorie intake from fats and achieving true ketosis can be quite daunting. From a food perspective, the high consumption of fatty and oily foods may be disgusting for many and can become incredibly boring after a while. If you follow a keto diet, you have to make an effort to ensure that you remain within the recommended daily carbohydrate intake. To achieve these levels, you must check nutrition labels to track your carbohydrate consumption. Why do math before you eat?

Another issue with the ketogenic diet is the consumption of foods containing high amounts of saturated fats. One should consume saturated fats in moderation, and they should not exceed 7% of a daily calorie intake. A diet high in saturated fat has been associated with increased low-density lipoprotein (LDL) cholesterol (the bad type), heart disease, and other cardiovascular-related issues. A meta-analysis, including 13 randomized controlled trials, assessed obese and overweight individuals for 1–2 years who followed either a low-fat diet or a very low-carbohydrate ketogenic diet. At the one year mark, the authors of the study found that the ketogenic diet achieved a 'small yet greater reduction' in triglycerides and blood pressure while increasing the amount of high-density lipoprotein (good cholesterol) and LDL cholesterol compared with participants who followed the low-fat diet.[8]

Since a ketogenic diet alters macronutrient composition (i.e., low carb, high fat), some studies were conducted to determine whether this truly affects weight loss. A narrative review, which included many meta-analyses, was done to assess the difference between a low-carbohydrate and low-fat diet in maintaining and achieving weight loss and whether one diet was superior to the other. The study authors wanted to ascertain whether there was an effect of macronutrient composition (quantity of carbohydrates or fat consumed) on weight loss.[57]

The study authors concluded that a lack of evidence offers no conclusion as to whether the low-carbohydrate or low-fat diet is superior to achieve or maintain weight loss.[57] One reason is the lack of a standard definition of 'low' fat or 'low' carbs. The American Academy of Physicians defines a low-carbohydrate diet as consuming <20% of carbohydrates.[40] The Atkins diet limits carbohydrate intake to 15–20 grams per day, especially during the beginning phase. Similarly, the definition of a 'low' fat diet remains ambiguous. Generally speaking, consuming <30% of calories from fat is considered a low-fat diet, and <20% of calories is considered a very low-fat diet.[4] With that, the authors said, "Without standard definitions, the idea that these diets could become universally prescriptive under any circumstances is unlikely." Also, to the authors' knowledge, there are no long-term studies looking at the macronutrient distribution on energy balance.

A meta-analysis including 13 randomized controlled trials evaluated whether participants following a very low carbohydrate ketogenic diet (VLCKD), comprising a diet of no more than 50g of carbohydrates per day, achieved 'better long-term body weight' compared to participants following a traditional low-fat diet (<30% of calories from fat). Authors found that the VLCKD achieved *short-term* effects on weight loss, yet the effects after one year in comparison to other common diets are not significantly different.[8]

Another meta-analysis of randomized controlled trials compared the effects of a low-carbohydrate diet ($\leq 45\%$ of calorie intake from carbs) versus a low-fat diet ($\leq 30\%$ of calorie intake from fat) on metabolic risk factors, body weight and waist circumference. Twenty-three trials, including a sample size of 2,788 participants from various countries across the globe, were included in the analysis as they met the inclusion criteria. The study authors found that 'low-carbohydrate diets are at least as effective as low-fat diets at reducing weight and improving metabolic risk factors.'[25]

In summary, if the amount of carbohydrates consumed is slightly modified, the general healthy population may experience health benefits and weight loss without having to go keto. Here's a reference for the ideal composition of a healthy plate of food:

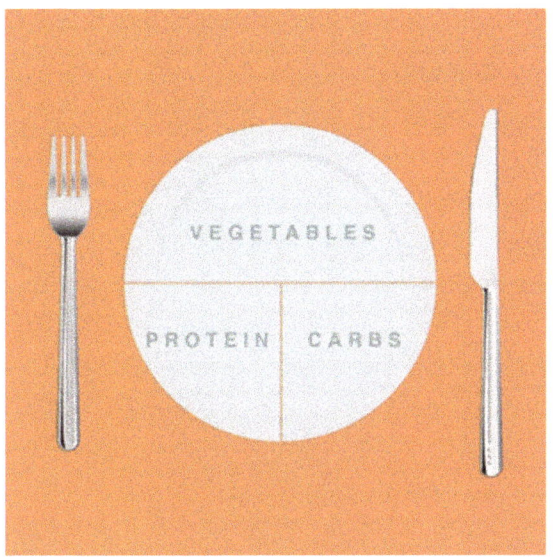

On the contrary, some studies suggest a benefit for weight loss when it comes to the ketogenic diet.[51] The reasons are:

- A high fat content may help suppress appetite and reduce sugar cravings.
- Ghrelin and leptin, appetite-stimulating hormones, are decreased as a result of a very low carbohydrate diet.
- Ketone bodies may help reduce hunger.

- Fat and protein require more energy expended when converted into glucose, hence increasing daily total energy expenditure.
- Fat loss is experienced due to the nature of the diet.

While these hold true, one may experience such benefits by eating regularly. There is no need to follow a keto diet to suppress your appetite. By focusing on consuming proteins, healthy fats, fiber and drinking water regularly throughout the day, you can experience a decrease in sugar cravings and suppress your appetite. With balanced eating, you can achieve this goal as effectively as the keto diet. Moreover, people who lose weight following a keto diet generally experience this due to water weight. As already mentioned, for every one gram of carbohydrate consumed, three grams of water is attached. Therefore, by reducing carbohydrate intake, there is a reduction in the attachment of water molecules, promoting weight loss to occur from water loss.

For the most part, the ketogenic diet is followed for medical reasons. Registered dietitian Kathy McManus, director of the Department of Nutrition at Harvard-affiliated Brigham and Women's Hospital, said, "The keto diet is primarily used to help reduce the frequency of epileptic seizures in children. We don't know if it works in the long term, nor whether it's safe."

Then comes the aftermath of the keto diet. Those who follow the diet and suddenly stop may indulge in carbohydrates. It causes them to retain more water and compensate by eating a high amount of carbohydrates, sugar, and calories; this leads to weight regain. The transition to come off of the keto diet requires careful planning. Aside from weight gain, those who don't plan their transition back to normal eating may experience other symptoms like bloating, increased hunger, sugar cravings and sugar spikes, leading to fatigue and irritability.

As a rule of thumb, here are three ways to smoothly transition off of a keto diet:

- **Focus on complex carbohydrates.** These carbohydrates don't cause a sudden spike in blood sugar levels as they take longer to digest than simple carbohydrates. Hence, focus on whole grains, legumes, and fibrous vegetables.
- **Gradually increase carbohydrate intake.** It's normal for someone to come off the keto diet and binge on ric, bread and pasta. The right way to transition from a keto diet is to increase carbohydrate intake gradually. A general rule is to increase your intake by around 10% per day.
- **Reduce sugar intake in the beginning.** It's best to avoid any sugary food which contains more than four grams of sugar. Keep the intake minimal at the start.

As you can see, the ketogenic diet does not qualify as a lifestyle diet. It's highly unsustainable to eat only fats, and it cuts out essential nutrients which come from fruits, vegetables, and carbohydrates. Some people might benefit from this diet; however, many others may experience hunger, irritability, mood swings, and constipation. While these symptoms may disappear, the keto diet presents other challenges, mainly the challenge of not enjoying your food. I love my carbs, and I'm sure you do too! So, following a keto diet, you can say goodbye to eating a delicious spaghetti bolognaise or some watermelon on a hot summer day.

A diet that is restricting and unenjoyable will eventually lead to dropout. Living this way is not sustainable, and it will most certainly lead to inconsistent eating patterns. After all, a lifestyle diet requires consistency to qualify it as a sustainable way of eating. Eliminating several food groups while experiencing challenges and side effects makes compliance difficult with the keto diet. It's why so many people can't go a very long time on the keto diet. They just can't tolerate all the oily, buttery and cheesy food anymore; they need their carbs, fruits and vegetables.

It all goes back to eating a balanced, varied, and healthy diet. If you couple this with good habits, you'll only feel great, and you'll be able to lose as much weight, if not more, than when following a ketogenic diet.

While the keto diet may help with weight loss, the results are equivocal. Most studies have looked at it for the short term (≤ 12 weeks), included a small sample size and lacked a control group. When designing studies, a control group is crucial to compare results to those not following a ketogenic diet. Additionally, more long-term studies are needed to understand the effects of the ketogenic diet on achieving and maintaining weight loss. Hence, the ketogenic diet does not qualify as a lifestyle diet.

"The easiest diet is, you know, eat vegetables, eat fresh food. Just a really sensible, healthy diet like you read about all the time."

—Drew Carey

Chapter 8
Plant-Based Diets

"Faisal, I need to lose weight. What do you think about going on a vegan diet?"

I cannot even count the number of times I have been asked this question.

Before I begin, I'd like to mention that I'm not against plant-based diets. For the vegans and vegetarians who follow a plant-based diet for ethical reasons (or any other reason for that matter), I am with you, and I respect your decision. No harm intended. I'm talking about switching to plant-based diets concerning *weight loss.*

Plant-based foods are excellent for your nutrition regimen. They offer numerous benefits, and I believe everyone should include a variety of plant-based foods in their daily nutrition. I actually like to dedicate 1–2 days a week (or several meals a week) to plant-based meals, purely for health reasons. However, my opinions, both personal and scientific, are around switching to plant-based eating specifically to lose weight. So please keep this in mind when reading this review.

Plant-based diets are all about eating foods derived from plants. Fruits, vegetables, nuts, seeds, whole grains, and legumes all fall under this diet. Typically, people following plant-based diets have concerns about animal treatment, the environment, a medical issue, or personal preference and taste. Sometimes, people follow a plant-based diet because of social pressure from family or friends.

There are variations of a plant-based diet, including:

- **Veganism.** Vegans eat no animal products. Therefore, honey, beeswax, gelatin, dairy, chicken, beef, fish, and eggs are not permitted.
- **Lacto-vegetarian.** This group includes dairy foods but still excludes eggs, beef, chicken, and seafood.
- **Ovo-vegetarian.** Only eggs are allowed here and no other animal products, including dairy.
- **Lacto-ovo-vegetarian:** This is the most common type of vegetarian diet. Lacto-ovo vegetarians consume egg and dairy products but exclude seafood, chicken, and beef.

Let me begin by talking about plant-based diets and weight loss. Here are three main reasons why I believe plant-based diets are not ideal for weight loss:

Consuming Excess Carbohydrates

Due to limited options, plant-based eaters can find themselves consuming large amounts of carbohydrates. For example, eating oatmeal for breakfast, a vegetarian pasta for lunch, some wheat crackers as a snack, and a vegan pizza for dinner are just way too many carbs, especially if you're sedentary. If excess carbs are consumed without being used for energy, the rest will be stored as fat. So unless you are tracking your intake, you may very well be eating more carbohydrates than you need, which will be a weight loss barrier.

Protein

It's essential to understand how different proteins are categorized. A protein's quality is determined by the protein digestibility-corrected amino acid score (PDCAAS). This score is based on the amino acid profile of proteins and their digestibility. The ability to digest protein matters because you essentially want to digest and absorb the protein from the food you eat efficiently.

We digest around 90–95% of the protein from animal-based foods, whereas our digestion rate for proteins from plant-based foods is between 60–80%. Therefore, we can digest and absorb more protein from animal-based foods, as figure 1 shows.[28]

Figure 1

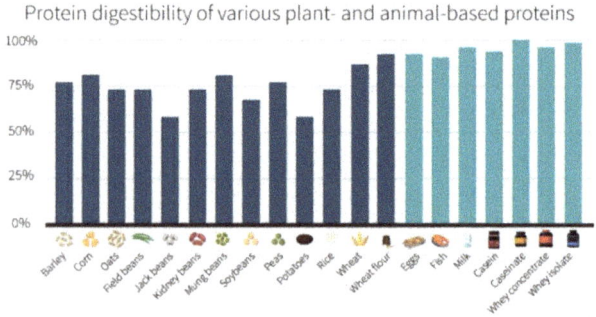

The second way to determine protein quality is by looking at its amino acid profile. The building blocks of protein are amino acids, and there are 20 amino acids in the body. Eleven of these are non-essential amino acids, meaning our body produces them. In contrast, nine are considered essential amino acids – so we need to get them through food because our body does not produce them.

As figure 2 shows, plant-based proteins contain less essential amino acids than animal proteins.[55,56] In particular, plant-based foods have a lower content of leucine, which is part of the three amino acids that make up BCAAs or branched chain amino acids. Leucine acts as a trigger to help muscles produce more protein.[67]

Figure 2

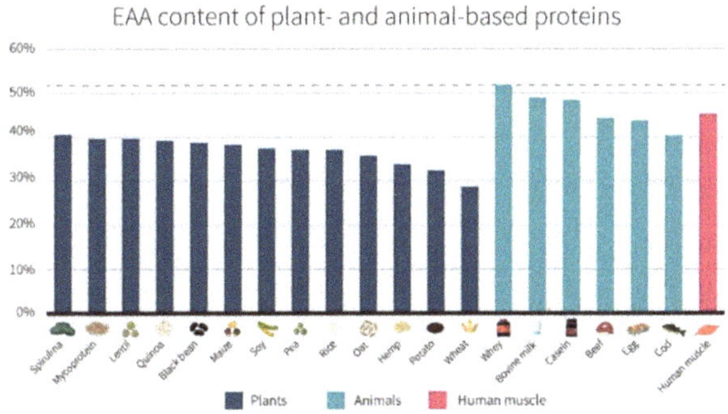

EAA content of plant- and animal-based proteins

An important nutrient for weight loss is protein. Protein suppresses appetite, which allows you to feel more satisfied throughout the day, helping you portion control and reduce your calorie intake. At the same time, protein has the highest thermic effect of food compared to carbohydrates and fat. The body burns around 20–30% of the calories consumed to digest and absorb protein, 0–3% of calories to digest fat, and 5–15% of calories to digest carbohydrates. Provided you are eating a protein-rich meal, 20–30% of the calories consumed are burned just to digest, absorb, and metabolize the protein. Thus, you're burning calories by simply eating protein.

What does this mean for plant-based diets? Well, aside from the fact that protein is digested and absorbed at a lower rate because plant-based proteins have a lower amino acid content and protein profile than animal-based proteins, those on plant-based diets also require a more significant amount and variety of plant-based proteins, namely chickpeas, lentils, beans, quinoa, chia seeds, nuts, and spirulina. Increasing the protein quantity means increasing the number of calories consumed. Again, to lose weight, one must be in a deficit. Since protein is an essential part of weight loss and those on their weight loss journey need to increase their protein intake, a higher protein consumption leads to higher calories per meal, slowing down the weight loss process.

For example, 100g of chicken breast contains around 27 grams of protein and 237 calories. In comparison, 100g of chickpeas contains 19 grams of protein and 364 calories (USDA). So you're getting less protein and more calories per meal.

A Low-Calorie Intake

Proponents of plant-based diets typically consume fewer calories than those on regular diets. The types of food included have a high fiber content and low-energy density, reducing daily calorie intake. At the same time, differences within plant-based diets exist. For example, those following a vegan diet generally consume fewer calories than other types of plant-based diets.

You can lose weight on a plant-based diet; it's just more complex and requires more effort. You can be vegan and lose weight, but if you're not controlling your portions and paying attention to what you eat, you may very well experience a weight increase. It would help if you were extremely meticulous with the composition of your meals, being sure to include 20–30 grams of protein per meal at the lowest calorie cost possible. Using mobile applications to help you track your food can be a good starting point until you get the hang of things.

Studies have shown a positive correlation between plant-based diets and weight loss.[12] Plant-based diets typically contain a good mix of fruits, vegetables, and whole grains. The low glycemic index values of vegetables and whole grains, coupled with the antioxidants, phytochemicals, minerals, and fiber found in fruit, have also demonstrated an inverse relationship between plant-based diets and weight loss.[24]

Like protein, fiber suppresses appetite; those who consume a diet high in fiber may feel more satisfied throughout the day, helping regulate hunger levels and sugar cravings. So those on a plant-based diet can experience weight loss. Additionally, fiber produces good bacteria in the gut (also referred to as probiotics), which helps with weight loss. When bacteria in the gut break down fiber, short-chain fatty acids are produced, decreasing the liver's triglycerides (fat in the blood).[12] It can also help regulate the production of hormones which contribute to hunger and fullness.

In a meta-analysis including 12 randomized controlled trials involving 1,151 subjects between the ages of 18–82, results found that those who followed a calorie-restricted vegetarian diet lost more weight than those in the non-vegetarian groups (average of 2.02kg weight-loss). Those on a vegetarian regimen also lost more weight (-2.12kg) than those who did not follow a calorie-restricted diet (-1.66kg).[26]

Now I know these studies contradict my point, but there are three things to realize. First, in relation to the meta-analysis, losing an average weight of 2.02kg is not significant. Second, other factors may have contributed to the weight loss other than just nutrition. For example, sleep, exercise, and other lifestyle factors impact your ability to lose weight. Third, while it appears that plant-based diets are indeed an effective weight loss intervention, we don't know the exact mechanism behind the weight loss experienced. One thing we do know, though, is an alternate in calorie balance. Plant-based eaters consume fewer calories than those following regular diets, which is needed to put the body in a calorie deficit to elicit weight loss.

You can still lose weight by maintaining a calorie deficit without following a plant-based diet. As highlighted in the meta-analysis, vegetarians following a *calorie-restricted* diet lost more weight than those following an unrestricted calorie diet. And that's how plant-based diets work.

While I am not undermining the power and benefit of plant-based diets, it all goes back to the basics of calories in versus calories out – the fundamentals behind weight loss is to burn more calories than you consume, plain and simple. If you are not a vegetarian, there is no need to completely change your lifestyle and follow a plant-based regimen to lose weight. Becoming a vegan or vegetarian will not accelerate the weight-loss process. Instead, you can eat a varied and balanced diet consisting of plant and animal-based foods and lose weight.

This is a segway into my final point on plant-based diets – the lifestyle element. Again, a lifestyle means living with balance – enjoying the foods you like, and eating all different kinds of food. Unless there are ethical or medical reasons for you to follow a plant-based diet, there is no need to restrict and limit yourself from so many foods and food groups purely to lose weight. If you love dairy, eat them. If you love chicken, beef, fish, and eggs, eat them too.

Plant-based diets are not magic for weight loss because you can still be in a calorie deficit and lose weight even if you incorporate animal-based food into your nutrition. For many, plant-based diets can be quite restricting and limiting, making it an unsustainable diet. For those reasons, plant-based diets are not deemed as a lifestyle diet.

"I don't believe in depriving myself of any food or being imprisoned by a diet."

—Joely Fisher

Chapter 9
The Paleo Diet

The Paleolithic diet, or the 'paleo' diet, is a diet which culminates the way human beings ate during the Old Stone Age – almost two million years ago. Life during this time was tough, and because of a lack of advanced tools, human beings used to hunt, fish, and gather wild plants for food. Proponents of this diet believe we should follow the way our ancestors used to eat during this time, as our genetics have not changed much since then. In addition, they believe a diet rich in lean meats and plant foods may help with diabetes, cancer and heart diseases, as our hunter-gatherer ancestors had reduced rates of these conditions because of their diet. In 2014, the paleo diet peaked, and it was during this time, people increased their desire to eat more healthily.[10]

The paleo diet consists of consuming lean meats, fish, fruits, vegetables, nuts, and seeds. Consuming foods high in protein, moderate in fat, low in carbohydrates, especially high-glycemic carbohydrates, and low in sodium and simple sugars are also permitted in the diet.[63] There is no 'true' paleo diet, as some people raised questions about food quality back then compared to today. For example, fruits and vegetables today do not resemble the quality of such produce during the

Stone Age. At the same time, do we know what foods actually existed during that period and what qualifies within the restrictions of a paleo diet? For example, white potatoes were readily available back then, but today, those on a paleo diet don't consume white potatoes as it is considered a high-glycemic carbohydrate.

Here is a quick summary of what the diet includes and excludes (we're back to limitations):

Includes: lean meats, fish (including shellfish), eggs, nuts, seeds, fruit, vegetables, avocado, olive oil, coconut oil, and vegetables.

Excludes: whole grains, cereals, dairy, white potato, legumes (mainly peanuts, beans, and lentils), coffee, salt, dairy, processed foods, and simple/added sugar (honey is okay but minimal quantities). Basically, these foods were not available to the hunter-gatherers during this era.

Now, onto the weight-loss and lifestyle discussion.

A 2015 systematic review and meta-analysis of four randomized controlled trials consisting of 159 participants compared the paleo diet with other dietary interventions on the short-term effects on waist circumference, triglycerides, blood pressure (systolic and diastolic), HDL cholesterol (the good type), and fasting blood sugar.[44]

The study did show the paleo diet to be short-term and more beneficial than other diets based on national nutritional guidelines. The paleo diet showed greater weight loss, reduced waist circumference, decreased blood pressure, improved cholesterol, and decreased insulin sensitivity. However, the studies included for review were short term (six months or less) and had small sample sizes (less than 40 participants in each study), so we can't make solid conclusions, especially regarding weight loss.[44] The authors of the study mentioned that more research needs to be done in this area, especially looking at the long-term benefits of the paleo diet and considering subjects' quality of life.

In a study conducted by Obert and others, they reviewed the epidemiology of obesity and popular fad diets and exercise programs that supposedly help with weight loss.[48] Among the fad diets was the Paleo diet, which led to weight loss due to *calorie restriction*. However, they found the studies on paleo diets to pose some limitations and basically put subjects on a calorie deficit – the fundamentals behind weight loss.

So, is the diet any special for weight loss? I'll let you answer that for yourself.

There are some downsides to the paleo diet, which does not qualify it as a lifestyle diet. First and foremost, the paleo diet is not feasible for everyone because it demands consuming fresh produce.[46] Lean, fresh meat and fish, and fresh produce are pricey, making it unaffordable for many people. Second, the authors of this study concluded that excluding food groups is also a limitation to maintaining this lifestyle for the long term.[46] Excluding food groups like whole grains and dairy increases the risk of micronutrient deficiencies, especially calcium, vitamin D, and B vitamins. Moreover, the decreased consumption of whole grains reduces fiber intake, which may increase the risk of diabetes and heart disease.[45] Legumes can also provide many nutritional benefits, mainly fiber, protein, iron, and copper, which are not allowed. In terms of the food included, a high intake of red meat can lead to a higher risk of diabetes, uric acid, and heart disease.

You may be wondering why our ancestors experienced better health markers through this way of eating. First, it's important to understand their levels of physical activity. Hunters and gatherers were way more active than we are today, and their food quality was significantly better. Hence, limitations of studies on the paleo diet included participants' quality of life, as this plays a vital role in understanding the health and weight-loss benefits of the diet.

Third, meal planning can be quite challenging. The paleo diet's heavy reliance on fresh foods means that followers of the diet need to plan, prepare, and cook their meals really carefully. The fast-paced world we live in today makes this difficult to adhere to. We barely have time to cut an apple, let alone purchase and cook fresh produce consistently. Due to the many restrictions with this diet, eating out at restaurants or social gatherings can make this even more challenging. You'd either have to bring your own food or make sure you know the exact ingredients in the food you're eating.

The paleo diet calls for eating whole and fresh foods while limiting processed foods, salt and added sugars. The exclusion of food groups like dairy and whole grains can lead to a suboptimal eating regimen. Additionally, financial and food preparation challenges make maintaining the paleo way of eating difficult. We also don't know if it's safe and beneficial for everyone, including the general healthy population and those at higher risks of certain diseases. Better quality studies with follow-ups of greater than one year are also needed to truly determine whether the paleo diet is indeed beneficial and superior to other dietary interventions.

In conclusion, the paleo diet is difficult to follow, and recommendations for weight loss by following a paleo diet can't be made just yet. Therefore, it is excluded as a lifestyle diet.

"Your diet is a bank account. Good food choices are good investments."
—Bethenny Frankel

Chapter 10
Detox Diets

Detox diets – the biggest scam and the ultimate fad diet, in my opinion.

If there's one diet I recommend you never even contemplate, it's a detox diet.

According to the Center for Disease Control and Prevention's Agency for Toxic Substances and Disease Registry, the definition of detoxification is 'the process of removing a poison or toxin or the effect of either from an area or individual.'

Mainstream detox diets aim to 'cleanse' and rejuvenate the body while helping eliminate any harmful toxins. Typical detox diets replace foods with liquids to cleanse your digestive system or enhance the body's detoxification system. In turn, you'll relax your digestive system, lose weight, and ultimately feel good. The most popular programs are juice cleanses, heavily restricted food intake, liver detoxification, and a colon cleanse.

There are a few things to note when it comes to detox diets. First, the body has its own detoxification system. Our liver, kidneys, lungs, and gastrointestinal tract constantly do the natural detoxing in your body. If you keep these organs strong and healthy, you'll enhance your body's detoxification system. Drinking green juices or herbal tea all day will not detox for you.

Second, the term 'toxins' remains ambiguous. In conventional medicine, 'toxins' typically refer to drugs and alcohol, and the detoxification process is weaning the body from such substances.[15] From a medical standpoint, detoxification occurs when the body excretes chemicals and their metabolism via urine or feces or extrarenal excretion through sweat or sebum.[37] Under scenarios such as drug overdose, high alcohol consumption and exposure to a toxic chemical, this can be done through injecting the body with charcoal. Typically, 25–100 grams of activated charcoal is injected into the body, which binds to the chemicals to prevent it from being absorbed in the gut and released into the bloodstream, eventually getting rid of these harmful substances via feces.[47,49]

Whereas the medical term for toxins is more precise, commercial detox programs' definition of toxins remains ill-defined. Most are unclear and revolve around pollutants, synthetic and heavy metals, processed food and other generally harmful products from modern-day life.[34]

Third, there are no specific toxins that we know of which are actually eliminated from the body. Most detox diets claim to help the body eliminate toxins without identifying which toxins are removed or the removal mechanism. In 2007, an investigative report, 'The Detox Dossier,' looked at the dodgy claims made by companies trying to promote detox products. The authors of the report examined 15 manufacturers who were promoting and distributing such products and wanted to know what the manufacturers meant by the word 'detox.'

"We discovered that companies often used phrases that sounded scientific but actually had little or no scientific meaning. We felt that the public was being duped. We wanted to do something about it and published our investigations with a call for other early career researchers to join us to Stand up for Science. And they did. They told us that there was more to be done, and the word that came up over and over again was DETOX. We all agreed that detox being used to sell everything from tea to hair straighteners was implausible and decided to dig deeper to find out what the product manufacturers meant by detox – had they some evidence about detox or how our bodies work not available to the rest of us? In fact, no one we contacted was able to provide any evidence for their claims or give a comprehensive definition of what they meant by 'detox.' We concluded that 'detox' as used in product marketing is a myth. Many of the claims about how the body works were wrong, and some were even dangerous."

Indeed, detox diets are nothing but a fad and remain ambiguous. Consumers are already confused about whether detox diets work or not, and even sellers seem confused. There is no uniform definition of what *detox* even means.

This does not mean that the body does not accumulate toxins. It does through the process of bioaccumulation. For example, we can be exposed to heavy metals like mercury from certain fish and toxins potentially found in protein powders.[38] Environmental persistent organic pollutants (POPs) are a type of toxicants stored in body fat. While our body fat can protect us from the short-term harmful effects of such a toxicant, with time, fat cells release POPs back into the system, increasing the risk of metabolic diseases.[29,39]

To date, no thorough studies have been conducted on detox diets. Furthermore, studies that have been published are poorly designed as they include a small sample size, lack control groups, incorporate a sample bias, and rely on self-reported and qualitative rather than quantitative measurements.[34]

The only clinically evaluated detox program is the Hubbard Purification Rundown, which conducted treatments to 14 rescue workers after being exposed to high levels of chemicals following the World Trade Centre collapse in 2001. The workers began to experience memory impairment after being exposed to polychlorinated biphenyls. The detoxification process entailed niacin supplementation, sweating in a sauna, and physical activity to remove stored toxins from fat cells. The rescue workers also took polyunsaturated oils, vitamins, minerals, and electrolytes to improve toxin excretion and support healing. Testing following this protocol showed improved scores on a memory test. However, due to the small sample size and no control group, conclusions cannot be drawn nor generalized from this study.[9]

There are not many studies to show the efficacy of detox diets when it comes to weight loss. In a study published in 2015, 84 pre-menopausal Korean women were divided into three groups: a control group without a diet restriction, a placebo group, and a lemon detox diet group. The placebo and detox group consumed 400 calories per day. The lemon detox program consisted of drinking a mixture of organic maple, palms, and lemon juice for seven days. The study authors looked at the program's effects on insulin sensitivity, inflammatory markers and anthropometric parameters such as weight and body fat. Results showed that both the detox and placebo groups lost weight and showed some health improvements; however, there wasn't a significant difference between the groups. The participants in both groups lost weight due to the calorie restriction.[36] If you consume 400 calories per day, of course, you'll lose weight.

Another study published in 2018 looked at the effects of a detoxification supplement on 22 young, healthy female adults. The organizers divided the participants into two groups, a placebo group, and a group taking the multi-ingredient detox supplement for four weeks. The supplement included '1,350 mg/serving of a proprietary blend of papaya leaf, cascara sagrada bark, slippery elm bark, peppermint leaf, red raspberry leaf, fenugreek seed, ginger root, and senna leaf.'[65] They analyzed body composition, waist circumference, symptoms of gastrointestinal distress, and several blood markers before and after supplementation. This study did not involve any calorie restriction; the authors found the detox supplement to have no significant effect on body composition or gastrointestinal symptoms.[65]

While some detox diet proponents will experience short-term weight loss, the weight loss experienced is due to a *calorie restriction* and not a magic detox program, pill or tea. You can also attribute any weight loss to a lack of carbohydrate consumption, which you already know is associated with more water loss, making up most weight loss on a detox diet. Still, some feel great when 'detoxing.' Generally, detox programs heavily restrict calories, remove problem foods (foods that may irritate the gut), and give rise to the placebo effect. In addition, if you're barely consuming calories from food, especially from protein, muscle loss will also comprise the weight loss experienced – which is not the right way to lose weight.

Depending on the detox program, some will advise removing specific food groups, like dairy. The dairy food group affects many, as a large percentage of the population is lactose intolerant; therefore, some people will feel great after removing these problematic foods (you'll soon find out that consuming dairy does pose health benefits). These cleansing diets are nothing more than an elimination diet, removing a particular food or food group to determine those that may potentially be problematic.

Furthermore, there are adverse health risks in undertaking detox diets. Due to the extreme calorie restriction, a lack of adequate nutrients, vitamin deficiencies, and electrolyte imbalances, even death can occur.[32] Also, those on detox diets may be at a greater risk of overdosing on supplements, laxatives, diuretics, and water.[34]

As with the supplement industry, detox programs are also not regulated. The lack of regulation makes detox diets a major concern and something you should consider carefully. In addition, there are reports that some companies are changing the words 'detox' and 'cleanse' to 'revamp' and 'reinvention,' making it more difficult to regulate detox diets and the industry as a whole.[34]

After all of this adverse information, how can you 'detox' the right way without having to try detox programs and potentially harm your health?

First, limit your exposure to airborne pollutants like smoke, smog, and chemical fumes by investing in proper air conditioning and ensuring that you have sufficient ventilation;

depending on where you live, wearing a face mask is important.

Second, enhance your liver's ability to detox for you. Cruciferous vegetables enhance the body's detoxification system as they contain a substance called sulforaphane.[35] These vegetables are called cruciferous vegetables because of their cross-shaped form and include broccoli, cauliflower, brussel sprouts, cabbage, arugula, kale, collards, watercress, and bok choy.

Third, keep smoked and chargrilled meats to a minimum, as cooking meats at high temperatures can damage the DNA and protein in our cells. I'm sure you've eaten a chicken breast or thigh which had burnt edges. If so, it's best to avoid the burnt edges as that's where the toxins are found. Stick to cooking methods which protect your meats from direct heat, such as steaming, poaching and stewing, and perhaps consider cutting the meat into smaller pieces to reduce the cooking time and high temperatures. If you were to eat charred meats, pair them with cruciferous vegetables to help eliminate the toxins more effectively. Additionally, cook meats with acidic-based marinades like lemon, lime, and vinegar.

Fourth, enhance your body's ability to remove toxins. Consuming a diet rich in fiber, especially soluble and fermented fiber, helps. Soluble fiber can bind to bile and toxins and help excrete them, while fermented fiber can feed and increase the good bacteria in the gut (acting like prebiotics). Prebiotics are essentially food for probiotics. Increasing the amount of good bacteria in the gut can help create short-chain fatty acids and other metabolites, which help the liver and kidney excrete toxins from the body.[14,68]

Another way to remove toxins is by sweating, and the best way to sweat is exercise.

While some detox programs advise a juice cleanse or liquid diet, the mere fact that you are sacrificing food consumption, which means nutrients, means you will lack the essential nutrients (vitamins and minerals) needed to keep your organs healthy and enhance the detoxification system. So rather than going on a calorie-restricted diet, liquid diet, or juice cleanse, to properly detox the body, you need to eat a well-balanced and varied diet – the basics of eating well.

Once again, all roads lead back to making healthy eating a *lifestyle* rather than sporadic dieting. Exercising, eating clean, whole and unprocessed foods, and shying away from airborne pollutants as best you can allow you to improve your health and well-being sufficiently for the body to carry the detoxification process on its own effectively. Drinking water throughout the day, keeping added sugar to a minimum, and giving your body the time to rest and recover are other things you can do to enhance your body's detox system.

There's no need to drink hot lemon water or celery juice all day. There's no need to drink detox teas. There's no need to be taking any supplements to detox. Instead, follow the basics of living a healthy lifestyle, which means eating well, sleeping well, and exercising, and you'll experience the beautiful benefits and detoxification which comes with it.

At present, there is no evidence suggesting that detox diets help with toxin elimination or weight loss. We don't know what toxins they actually remove, and the short-term weight loss experienced is due to a calorie restriction, as usual. Hence, it does not qualify as a lifestyle diet.

"I don't go long without eating. I never starve myself."
—Vanessa Hudgens

Chapter 11
Intermittent Fasting

Intermittent Fasting (IF) is another buzz diet of the past few years and probably the most popular diet today. Intermittent fasting gained popularity in 2012 after Dr. Mosely, a BBC journalist, created a documentary called *Eat, Fast and Live Longer* and published a book, *The Fast Diet*. In 2013, Kate Harrison published a book, *The 5:2 Diet,* which further increased the popularity of IF.

Intermittent fasting is all about planning and timing *when* you eat instead of planning *what* you should be eating. It's not your typical diet of eliminating certain foods or food groups or placing other limitations on what you eat; it's more of an eating pattern.

History tells us that IF has been practiced before. Hunters and gatherers went through long periods without food – they weren't privileged with supermarkets to purchase food when needed or refrigerators to store their food. During specific periods, religions such as Islam, Christianity, Judaism, and Buddhism practice intermittent fasting. Consequently, humans have evolved and adapted to survive prolonged periods without food.

You can practice intermittent fasting in many ways. Some prefer the conventional pattern of fasting for 16 hours and eating during an 8-hour window. Others prefer to fast for 12 hours and eat in a 12-hour window, while many prefer eating regularly and fasting for 24 hours straight, one or two days a week. There's no standard method. It's more about developing an eating pattern, and many may play around with the hours, finding an option to suit their lifestyle. One of the most popular patterns is the 5:2 diet, whereby five days of the week are regular eating days, while the remaining two days see a restriction in calories to 500 per day.

Intermittent fasting does pose benefits to our body and overall health. For example, studies have shown IF to improve insulin resistance by helping decrease blood sugar levels by 3–6% and insulin by 20–31%, both of which can help prevent type 2 diabetes.[5] By decreasing insulin resistance, the body increases its insulin sensitivity, meaning glucose is more efficiently transferred from the bloodstream into the cells (since the pancreas releases insulin to transfer sugar in the blood into the cells). Improving insulin sensitivity helps regulate the body's blood sugar levels, avoiding sudden spikes or crashes.

Intermittent fasting also improves the body's fat-burning capacity – not necessarily aiding fat loss but rather helping the body adapt to burning fat as fuel. Moreover, IF can improve brain health; it may help with certain diseases like Alzheimers and Parkinsons by increasing the production of brain-derived neurotrophic factor (BDNF), helping with the growth of new nerve cells.[16,22] However, more studies need to be conducted on humans to warrant a relationship between IF and brain health, as most current studies have been done on animals.

Studies have also shown intermittent fasting to reduce inflammation in the body. Some inflammation is needed to fight infections, as inflammation triggers certain chemicals which help reduce the inflammation itself. However, chronic inflammation can be detrimental to our health and well-being, as studies have linked it with certain conditions like heart diseases and rheumatoid arthritis.[27] A cross-sectional study was conducted on 51 healthy subjects to investigate the effects of intermittent fasting during Ramadan on certain inflammatory and immune biomarkers. During Ramadan, Muslims fast between sunrise and sunset – very similar to the 16/8 hour fasting method. The study authors analyzed these health markers one week before Ramadan, at the end of the 3rd week of Ramadan, and one month after Ramadan had ended. The study found that pro-inflammatory blood markers were reduced during Ramadan as opposed to before or after.[17]

Furthermore, a study showed that intermittent fasting improves heart health by improving blood pressure, triglycerides, and cholesterol levels. In a study conducted in 2007, 110 obese subjects were hospitalized for three weeks to treat their obesity with the fasting diet. Before, during and after the study, the authors analyzed blood pressure, total cholesterol, triglyceride levels, and other health parameters and found a significant decrease in these areas.[6]

Intermittent fasting poses many health benefits. Considering this way of eating depends on how you feel when fasting, how convenient it is for you, whether you enjoy it or not, and whether you can actually sustain this eating pattern.

Overweight and obesity is a global health concern due to the lack of physical activity and overconsumption of foods, especially energy-dense foods.[53] The most common method of treatment is daily calorie restriction, which many people find challenging. For this reason, intermittent calorie restriction was developed, including a 'feed' day, to consume food *ad libitum* for 24 hours, and a 'fast' day, restricting food intake for 24 hours.[66] This pattern of eating, also known as alternate day fasting, seemed to increase compliance and adherence.

While both daily calorie restriction and alternate-day fasting have been tested to see whether they elicit a weight-loss response, the understanding of which method produced superior weight-loss and body composition improvements was yet to be determined. Hence, a study was conducted comparing these two eating methods on weight loss, fat mass loss, muscle mass retention and visceral fat mass in overweight and obese adults. Studies in this review had to meet the following criteria, i) randomized control trials, ii) studies which looked at weight loss and body composition changes, iii) daily calorie restriction and alternate-day fasting as the main intervention methods used and analyzed, iv) study duration of 4–24 weeks, v) adult populations, vi) overweight or obese participants, and vii) non-diabetic subjects.[66]

The study found a similar degree of weight loss with alternate-day fasting as with daily calorie restriction. Short-term study results (3 to 12 weeks) showed alternate-day fasting to reduce body weight from baseline by around 4–8%, whereas daily calorie restriction showed a 5–8% reduction. Not entirely significant. Regarding fat mass, trials lasting 8–12 weeks showed an 11–16% decrease through alternate-day fasting and a 10–20% reduction through daily calorie restriction.[66] Again, not a significant difference.

Visceral fat mass was also analyzed. Visceral adipose tissue is located in the abdominal cavity and between organs (liver, kidneys, stomach, intestines, etc.). It is referred to as organ fat or abdominal fat. The review showed that visceral fat was reduced by 4–10% through alternate-day fasting and 6–13% through daily calorie restriction.[66] Again, not a significant variance.

An interesting finding highlighted the notion of alternate-day fasting being the better option to retain lean muscle mass than daily calorie restriction. Those following the alternate-day fasting lost around 90% of their weight from fat, and 10% as fat-free mass, whereas those who followed the daily calorie restriction protocol lost 75% of their weight from fat and 25% as fat-free mass.[66]

What's the point here? While studies have shown intermittent fasting to be safe and effective for weight loss, it's no different from following a balanced eating pattern, including daily calorie restriction. You can still lose weight by putting your body in a daily calorie deficit without having to go through periods of fasting.

When you skip meals to reduce calories, you will lose weight – that's why many people consider IF for weight loss. But with fasting comes muscle loss, and depending on compliance, it may lead to an extreme calorie deficit, which, as I've alluded to many times already, can cause health problems and even reverse the weight-loss process. Intermittent fasting is not a one-way ticket to weight loss. Bear in mind, the initial weight loss experienced is due to water loss, but after returning to regular eating, the weight lost (and more) can potentially be regained. Sorry to burst your bubble, but this weight gain will be in the form of fat, not muscle.

Based on my experience with clients who practice intermittent fasting, they barely meet their caloric needs during their window of eating. Since they are hungry, their first meal is typically heavy and filling. In addition, some find it difficult to consume 3–4 meals during an eight-hour window. Without a structured eating pattern, you may put your body into a large calorie deficit, leading to a slower metabolism and a decreased ability to lose weight if followed for an extended period. After an extended fast, many also tend *not* to focus on the quality of their food and justify an unhealthy (cheat) meal, so there is also a psychological effect. People think they deserve to eat a heavy and greasy meal after fasting all day. The quantity and quality of your food are equally important. Whether intermittent fasting or reducing daily calorie intake, consuming poor-quality food can backfire. Some will eat more than one meal during their eating window, but because they may choose energy-dense (high calorie) meals, they may very well be in a calorie surplus, which will lead to weight gain.

If you were to follow intermittent fasting, I can't stress enough the importance of following a sound and structured nutrition plan because it is very easy to do it incorrectly and hinder the weight-loss process. To reap the benefits of intermittent fasting, you have to nail your eating window and be meticulous about your timing and food composition.

From a lifestyle perspective, no one fasts forever or for very long periods because it's simply not sustainable. Hence, in my opinion, IF is not deemed as a lifestyle diet. It will provide short-term solutions and quick fixes, as do most other diets, but more research is needed for longer-term interventions, including adherence to this approach to eating. It's essential to find a way of eating which is convenient, sustainable and enjoyable to you. If intermittent fasting does not tick one of these boxes, then I'd advise against it. Fasting is not for everyone. Those who are underweight or have a history of eating disorders should not follow this eating pattern.

While intermittent fasting does provide health benefits, it can also be dangerous; some people experience dizziness, headaches, low blood sugar, muscle soreness, and fatigue. If not structured well, longer-term fasting can also lead to anemia, a weakened immune system, and vitamin and mineral deficiencies. For some, fasting makes them feel more comfortable, reduces their hunger, helps them lose weight, helping them feel good overall. Others may feel very uncomfortable with increased hunger and sugar cravings, keeping them feeling tired and lethargic all day.

From an exercise perspective, if you train every day and practice intermittent fasting, you may risk losing the energy and calories you need to perform and recover at optimal levels. If you feel strongly about following this eating pattern, I highly recommend planning your exercise sessions during your eating window. At least you can eat before, during and after your exercise session for enhanced performance and recovery.

The bottom line: intermittent fasting can benefit our health and wellbeing if done right and for a short period. It can also lead to short-term weight loss. However, from a weight-loss perspective, it doesn't greatly differ from eating throughout the day and maintaining a daily calorie deficit.

From a lifestyle perspective, it's simply not sustainable. So, to fast or not to fast? That is the question I'll leave you to answer.

"Creating an overall healthy lifestyle for yourself doesn't require a radical diet or significant life change. In fact, it can be attained through common sense decisions about the way we eat, move, and live."
—Harley Pasternak

Chapter 12
Study Findings and Expert Opinions

Take a second and absorb everything you've now read about some of the most popular diets.

What do you think of them? Are they fad diets? Do they work? Is this how you want to eat for the rest of your life?

Medical reasons aside, it's evident that diets are nothing more than trends, and when it comes to weight loss, they're not magic.

Many have conducted studies to compare different diets and their effect on weight loss. Johnston and colleagues reported findings from a range of meta-analyses which looked at the effectiveness of popular diets on weight loss and the availability of published data from randomized control trials. Network meta-analysis can help manage expectations when choosing one diet over the other by standardizing analyses such that the commercial diet vendors themselves do not influence them.

The study included 48 randomized control trials, 43 of which reported weight loss at six months, and five trials reported weight loss at 12 months. The study authors concluded that low carbohydrate and low-fat diets led to a loss of around 8kg at six months and 6–7kg at 12 months if compared with no diet.[30]

While this review is credible given the research strategy, eligibility criteria for study selection and data extraction system, the study's authors believe the study's limitations are important to consider. When analyzing studies which focus on moderate macronutrient consumption, authors found such studies to be involved with food replacement products, different behavioral approaches, and other differences, making it difficult to compare one diet with another. At the same time, a sensitivity analysis was not conducted to better understand the level of adherence to the different diets and whether the level of adherence or the diet composition itself was the reason behind the weight loss.[30]

Another randomized control trial was conducted, otherwise known as the Preventing Overweight Using Novel Dietary Strategies (POUNDS LOST), which assessed differences in weight-loss through four different approaches: (1) a low-fat, average protein diet (20% fat, 15% protein, and 65% carbohydrate), (2) a low-fat, high protein diet (20% fat, 25% protein, and 55% carbohydrate), (3) a high-fat, average protein diet (40% fat, 15% protein, and 45% carbohydrate), and (4) a high-fat, high protein diet (40% fat, 25% protein, and 35% carbohydrate). Unsurprisingly, at the two-year mark, weight loss was similar across all diets. Abdominal fat, body fat, and hepatic (liver) fat were the same, with no differences in lean muscle mass.[13]

Another study served as a follow-up to the above trial, investigating whether the fat and protein content of the four different diets analyzed affected food cravings in overweight and obese adults. While there were some short-term differences in the two years, a sample of 811 participants showed that weight loss occurred due to decreased cravings for fats, sweets, and starches, while cravings increased for fruits and vegetables. The authors also found that calorie-restricted diets (regardless of the macronutrient distribution) led to these changes in cravings. The authors concluded that weight loss occurs successfully by maintaining a calorie deficit while adhering to the diet.[3]

Taking a slightly different approach than addressing well-conducted studies, I'd like to share the insights on diets and weight loss from some of the best scientists and practitioners in the field of nutrition and exercise.

Let me begin by sharing an excerpt from a blog post written by Asker Jeukendrup. Asker is one of my favorite researchers and practitioners in the realm of nutrition, especially within sports and exercise performance. He has over 30 years of experience as a researcher, practitioner, and consultant. He has published over 200 peer-reviewed studies and book chapters and published several books himself. Credible individual? Most definitely. Here's what he has to say about diets for weight loss:

"Many will talk about the 'type' of weight that is lost and I can certainly agree that fat loss should most often be emphasized over lean (muscle) loss and it appears pretty clear that high(er) protein and exercise (particularly resistance exercise) are effective in this regard. But the fundamental truism is that E (energy/calorie) balance has to be negative and when you do that, and can sustain your new weight (likely by following the same approach you used to lose it), then you achieve success! But as we know, the success rate of weight loss is not good (yes, that's an understatement), and yet every dietary bestseller and concept that comes out has a new theory as to what it is that causes weight/fat gain and how to reverse it 'Forever' and to 'Forget everything you've ever been told' or that 'What you've heard is all wrong.' I don't doubt that there's a shred of truth in everyone's approach, but Ockham's razor would suggest that there's a really simple truth behind all weight loss programs, and it really has to be whether you can stick to staying in negative energy balance to lose the weight and then stick to your new energy intake, eating less, forever...which as we know is a long time! So stick to it is what wins? Well, I think that's a big part of it."

Professor Stuart Phillips, a Tier 1 Canada Research Chair and professor in the Department of Kinesiology and School of Medicine at McMaster University, said, "The fundamental truism is that energy balance has to be negative and when you do that, and can sustain your new weight, then you achieve success!"

In an interview by Predator Nutrition with nutrition and fitness experts, some of the most influential figures in the field expressed their opinion on diets and fat loss. Alan Aragon, an influential figure with over 20 years of experience in the fitness field and who has been pushing the movement toward evidence-based information, said, "The most important thing is to sustain a caloric deficit over a prolonged period. The deficit will periodically close up, and plateaus in fat loss will occur, and getting past those plateaus is a matter of re-opening the deficit with either a further decrease in intake, increase in training output, or both."

Layne Norton, a renowned physical preparation and physique coach with a Ph.D. in Nutritional Sciences, said,

"Well, there are a lot of things, but the biggest thing is to make sure that you are in a caloric deficit. Obviously, protein, carb, and fat breakdown is going to heavily influence substrate utilization, and exercise is important to maintain muscle mass, but at the end of the day, if you aren't oxidizing more than you take in, you won't be seeing a significant fat loss in most cases."

Borge Fagerli, a teacher at the Academy for Personal Training (AFPT) and inventor of Myo-Reps™, said, "I would say consistency. It's not usually a matter of the diet failing the dieter; it's the dieter failing the diet. When things start to slow down, which it inevitably does on any diet when you get into low single-digit BF% (body fat), is when you need a hefty dose of patience to stick it out. And by that, I'm not only talking about binge eating episodes; I'm talking about being over-ambitious and cutting calories harder or adding cardio to an already borderline excessive deficit. Trust the process and make sure you have sufficient nutrients to not only maintain training intensity but to function in daily life. Take your time. If you're always hungry and obsessed with food, you should seriously consider adding calories or changing your macros around – unless you're at the very end of a contest diet where some suffering is bound to happen, of course…"

Matt Lovell, a sports nutritionist with experience working in elite sports such as the English Premier League as a nutrition consultant with Tottenham Hotspurs and Manchester City Football Clubs, said, "Find a balance which you can stick to which contains the right mix of deficit, muscle protection, nutrient delivery and sustainable longer-term adherence."

The evidence suggests that diets do not work; they are no better than eating regularly while ensuring you maintain a daily calorie deficit.

As you can see from the studies mentioned and the opinions of renowned practitioners and researchers in the field, it's crucial to interpret the research when reading it and scrutinize the diet itself. Many factors impact weight loss other than macronutrient distribution (i.e., low fat, low carb, etc.). Adherence, nutrient quality, lifestyle choices, and calorie balance are among the many factors that impact a diet's success in weight loss.

Should you diet for weight loss? Absolutely not! You are wasting your time and actually causing more harm than good. As I mentioned repeatedly, you can still eat in a balanced way, enjoy your food, put your body in a daily calorie deficit, and lose weight. There's no need to starve or deprive yourself, remove any foods or food groups you enjoy, and put yourself through the physical, mental and emotional struggle which comes with dieting. Life is too short to live this way.

What is the best diet? It's the one you can stick to. How can you be consistent with the diet you choose to follow? By enjoying the foods you eat. This is my view and the view of so many other researchers and practitioners in the field. Unfortunately, this advice is not what the general public likes to hear, but it's a fact.

People listen to people – this is the unfortunate truth of human beings today. If an influencer on social media promotes their routine, others will blindly implement this in their lives (and then get frustrated because of a lack of results). If someone invents a diet for the sake of exploiting others for their financial benefit, people will follow. If I tell my social media followers, "Don't eat tomatoes at night because it will make you fat," I guarantee many will take this advice wholeheartedly and implement it.

I'm not trying to be condescending; I'm stating the scientific truth. This is why it's essential to do your due diligence, research the diet you are contemplating, and know more about the person behind the information. Not everyone is qualified or credible to address people's health issues, so be mindful of the source of your information.

Overall, diets do not work and are merely a waste of time, effort, and money. Findings of studies and opinions from *credible* and *qualified* scientists and practitioners in the field emphasize the importance of effective lifestyle interventions which promote habit and behavioral changes, adherence and compliance to a *calorie-restricted* diet, eating nutrient-dense foods, and following a balanced eating regimen. Don't diet. Make it a lifestyle.

"The heart, like the stomach, wants a varied diet."
—Gustave Flaubert

Chapter 13
Fact or Fad?

Can we now agree that diets don't work? The purpose of writing this book is to prove this point, and I hope to have now convinced you never to contemplate going on a diet again.

Science says it all. I've shared high-quality studies, insights from scientists and experts and simply laid out the *facts*.

I'll revisit the point I made at the beginning of this book – please do not give into all the noise surrounding diets, including what Instagram influencers, Netflix documentaries, and people with one nutrition 'certification' tell you. Science has shown you; diets do not work.

What conclusions can you draw from the diets I've highlighted? If there's one common message, it's that they all remove specific foods or food groups from your diet. Indeed, this is one paramount quality of a *fad* diet.

Now that you have a basic understanding of today's most trendy diets, the next step is to educate you on how to detect fad diets on your own. It is important because once you have the tools, you'd be better equipped to analyze if a diet is a fad or based on science, and better yet, start to appreciate the true meaning of healthy eating as a lifestyle.

It's simple to find diets online. Just type the word 'diet' on Google, and you'll find so many trendy diets with no solid evidence behind them.

Numerous diets are promoted as being the best or the only way to lose weight. Some restrict calories to the extreme, some eliminate essential nutrients, and some eliminate entire food groups. Any diet which does one of these three things is essentially a fad diet.

For example, fad diets might include low-carb, high-fat, or high protein. Some focus on specific foods, like cabbage or animal meats, while others focus on eating at specific times of day only.

Whatever the diet requirements may be, all fad diets have one thing in common: a quick and temporary solution to what has been a lifelong problem to many people.

Before I provide you with ways to detect fad diets, it's vital to ask yourself questions before trying any new diet.

Can you follow a strict diet? Have you ever tried a diet before? If you did, how did you feel mentally, physically, and emotionally? It's really important to understand your personal needs and experiences before you consider following any diet.

While there is no standard approach to spotting a fad diet, there are some red flags. Here are eight ways to spot a fad diet:

1. Approaches Which Recommend a Quick Fix.

Any diet or challenge that promises you to lose a certain amount of weight in a short period is complete nonsense.

Losing weight in a short period is unhealthy, and you'll definitely regain the weight faster than you lost it.

2. Statements That Are Over the Top.

Many diets make claims on the amazing benefits and results you'll experience once you start their diet. Anything that sounds too good to be true probably is, so don't even bother with it. There are no magic diets. For example, if you see a claim saying, 'lose 20 lbs. in 20 days,' then you know it's undoubtedly a fad diet.

3. Advice Based on a Single Study.

Any diet which makes claims based on a single study is a fad diet. To draw a solid conclusion requires evidence backed by numerous studies. This is why I've provided you with evidence based on systematic reviews and meta-analyses. A systematic review uses a systematic method to answer specific research questions by gathering all available empirical research. A meta-analysis analyzes and combines various results from similar studies using a statistical process.

4. A List of Good and Bad Food.

There is no such thing as good or bad food. We all have different preferences. What might be good for one person may be bad for another, and vice versa. If a diet includes a list of good and bad foods, ignore it because it's a fad diet.

5. Recommendations to Sell a Product.

Any diet associated with a product, like supplements, pills, or teas, is a red flag and a sign of a fad diet. The creator of the diet is looking to exploit you to make money.

6. Drawing Conclusions from Studies Which Are Not Peer-Reviewed.

Peer-reviewed studies are when other experts in the field review a study before it's published. Any study that is not peer-reviewed yet makes claims about a specific diet should be ignored. Do your research!

7. Studies Ignoring Differences Between Individuals and Groups.

Everyone is different. It's not a one size fits all approach. A diet based on studies which generalize claims without considering differences among individuals and groups is a fad diet.

8. Elimination of One or More Food Groups.

If a diet eliminates either fruits, vegetables, fats, carbohydrates, or protein, then you know it's a fad diet for sure. Eating in a balanced way by incorporating all food groups is the best way to make healthy eating a lifestyle.

It is very tempting to follow a diet to lose weight in the shortest time possible; you should know that serious health issues are associated. Not only will fad diets slow down your metabolism, but they can also lead to eating disorders, dehydration, digestive problems, and even malnutrition, which basically means depriving your body of the essential nutrients it needs to survive and function at its best.

Fad diets have been around for a long time, and while their names or approaches are changing, you need to be wary of them. You mainly need to be aware of anything that offers a quick fix.

To help with your research, here are some of my favorite websites and Instagram accounts to follow, which provide high-quality scientific information:

Websites

www.precisionnutrition.com
www.examine.com
www.webmd.com
www.mayoclinic.com
www.harvardhealth.com

Instagram accounts

@precisionnutrition
@examinedotcom
@edible_evidence
@thealanaragon
@dietetically_speaking
@martinnutrition

"There's no quick or magical way to lose weight. You just have to do it the natural way and be able to do it on your own pace."

—Jordin Sparks

Chapter 14
Debunking Nutrition Myths

Take a second and think about some of the nutrition statements you've heard or read before. Did you ever do your own research to ensure that it's a fact?

The problem with today's world, especially with social media, is sharing information without a scientific basis. We sometimes don't even know the source of this information and whether or not they have the right background and appropriate qualifications to be advising people on their health.

With the information overload, we don't know what's right or wrong anymore. One day, we hear dairy is good for us; the next day, we hear dairy is bad for us. I don't blame you for feeling more confused and frustrated than ever before.

Well, don't worry. I'm here to debunk some nutrition myths and make sure we silence the noise.

There's so much nutrition information on the internet, and the problem is that so much of it is inaccurate. Let me share some nutrition facts so that you feel more confident about your food choices. There are many myths to debunk, but I'll discuss eight of the most common.

1. Avoid Carbs After 7 PM.

This one just blows my mind. A lot of people think avoiding carbs at night is a good strategy to lose weight. Firstly, your body doesn't even know when it's 7 pm. Secondly, weight loss occurs from being in a calorie deficit and not about the timing of when you eat carbs. So don't worry, there is absolutely nothing wrong with eating carbs at night. As long as you are in a daily calorie deficit, you will lose weight.

2. A Detox Diet Will Cleanse My Body from Toxins.

You now know that there is little evidence to substantiate the claimed benefits of detox diets. Your lungs, kidneys, and gastrointestinal tract will do the detoxing in your body for you. It's not about a juice cleanse or fasting for 16 hours. As long as you keep your lungs, kidneys, and gut healthy, your body will detox automatically and efficiently.

3. Dairy Is Bad for You.

I get it. Many media outlets and organizations have painted dairy in a negative light, causing an increased skepticism toward the consumption of dairy products. I can assure you that there is nothing wrong with dairy. Unless you are allergic, lactose intolerant, or experience a bad reaction when consuming dairy, there is absolutely nothing wrong with incorporating dairy into your nutrition plan. Like anything else, you should have nothing to worry about if consumed in moderation. Let me expand more on this as this is a hot topic.

Dairy is quite beneficial. In 2016, Thorning and colleagues presented a narrative review assessing the scientific evidence from meta-analyses of observational studies and randomized control trials which looked at the relationship between dairy consumption and risk of obesity, type 2 diabetes, cardiovascular diseases, osteoporosis, cancer, and all-cause mortality.[64]

The studies found that the consumption of milk and dairy products was correlated with a reduced risk of obesity in children while improving body composition and facilitating weight loss in adults during a calorie restriction. It also found that consuming 200–300ml of milk does not increase the risk of cardiovascular disease. In fact, there was an inverse relationship shown between the consumption of dairy products with hypertension and stroke.[64] In terms of bone health, a positive effect was shown between dairy products on bone health in childhood and adolescence, although limited evidence was found of this relationship in adults and on the risk of bone fractures in older age.

According to the World Cancer Research Fund (WCRF) and meta-analyses, they found milk and dairy products protective against colorectal, bladder, gastric, and breast cancer. While the evidence for prostate cancer is limited, dairy products do not seem to be associated with the development of pancreatic, ovarian, or lung cancer.[64]

Finally, the relationship between the consumption of dairy products and 'all-cause mortality' (all-causes of death) has also been highlighted. Based on meta-analyses of observational cohort studies, evidence in the literature does not suggest that the consumption of dairy products is associated with all-cause mortality.[64]

So, got milk?

4. Gluten Is Bad for You

Similar to dairy, there is nothing wrong with eating gluten when considering a clinically healthy population. Unless you have Coeliac disease or gluten intolerance, you shouldn't worry about considering a gluten-free lifestyle.

There are many publicized benefits of a gluten-free diet. Yet, there are links to this particular diet and changes in healthy gut microbiota, production of short-chain fatty acids, disordered eating, and a compromised energy and nutrient intake.[23,59]

Whether you go on a gluten-free diet by choice or dictated by medical treatment, you should be guided by an appropriate diagnosis and dietary management to reduce the risk of overlooking the primary causes and unnecessary food restriction.[11,23,59]

5. Eating at Night Will Make Me Fat.

Like the carbs situation, it's not eating at night that will make you fat; it's a calorie surplus that will make you fat. If you are consuming more calories than you are burning, you will gain fat. Eating too late at night and sleeping right after can delay digestion, and you may wake up feeling bloated and heavy. But in terms of weight loss, it's down to a calorie balance. Don't worry; you can enjoy a nice and healthy snack at night if you're hungry.

6. So Long as I Exercise, I Can Eat Whatever I Want.

You go to the fast-food drive through a couple of times a week, you fill your grocery cart with chips, cookies, and sweets, and you exercise every day. You're thin, and you don't seem to gain weight. So everything is good, right?

Not really.

Try not to use exercise as an excuse to overeat. Thinking that you need to exercise more or exercise harder to give yourself that leeway to enjoy burgers and pizzas every day is not the best idea, and won't form a healthy relationship with food. You can't outrun a bad diet. No matter how much you exercise, you won't experience the many benefits if you are eating unhealthily.

Suppose you're exercising every day, eating whatever you want, and the number on the scale seems healthy. Does this mean you're healthy too? No, you have to realize that while exercise is really important during your health journey, it is not the be-all-end-all. For optimal health, you need to approach it holistically, focusing on eating well, exercising well, sleeping well, managing stress, and adopting positive habits.

People think they can eat whatever they want based on the simple fact that they burn more calories by exercising and believing they have more flexibility to eat cheat-like meals. It's much easier to consume calories than it is to burn calories. We tend to overestimate the number of calories we burn and underestimate the number of calories we consume. At the same time, the quality of your food will directly impact the quality of your exercise; it is best to be eating the right type of food to gain the best from your exercise. Hence, the recommendation is to move more and eat less. Not necessarily eating less to the point of deprivation, but focusing on consuming nutrient-dense foods and limiting your intake of calorie-dense foods.

There is a mental catch-22 between food and exercise. Many say, "I eat well when I exercise. It's when I don't exercise that I eat poorly." By exercising, we subconsciously start eating better. Changing our lifestyle and exercising makes us feel the need to eat properly. But then suddenly, something happens, and we have to stop exercising. From here, eating and food choices just go downhill.

It's of utmost importance to try and eat well the majority of the time, not only when you exercise.

Eating healthy shouldn't be seasonal; it should be all year round whether you exercise or not. This is what it truly means to live a healthy lifestyle – you're practicing these healthy habits, every day, of every week, of every month, of every year. If you can't outrun a bad diet, then do you really believe you can sustain not eating well when you don't exercise? Some food for thought. Exercise and nutrition in combination will boost your health and well-being. Bridge the two, and you'll feel so much better.

7. Superfoods Will Keep You Super Healthy.

Superfood is a buzzword you've probably seen on products, in health stores and written about in many blog articles and social media posts. It seems like every year we discover a new superfood. Goji berries, kale, chia seeds – the list goes on. While the claimed superfoods are healthy foods to incorporate in your nutrition plan, there aren't any foods that will cure cancer or make you lose weight. Most superfoods are a hype and built off of the next trend without any magic health benefits or substantial evidence to back them up.

While there is no such thing as a 'superfood,' there are four foods backed by solid evidence supporting their benefits: garlic, spirulina, berries, and leafy greens.

As you know, one way to detect a fad diet is if its claim is too good to be true. Most superfoods, especially new ones we hear of, are almost always too good to be true. Please don't rely on social media, influencers, or products to show you new discoveries of foods and their powerful benefits. As usual, do your homework and rely on changing your habits to live healthily rather than focusing on incorporating 'superfoods' into your nutrition.

8. You Need to Take Multivitamins to Remain Healthy.

Vitamins and minerals are considered 'micronutrients' because we need them in small quantities to satisfy our daily needs. If you're eating a variety of fruits and vegetables daily, then you won't need to use any multi-vitamins because you'll be satisfying your micronutrient intake.

I hope I've helped you feel better by debunking some ridiculous statements we hear time and time again. It's vital to do your due diligence and research topics independently from trusted websites and credible practitioners to separate the myths from the facts. Doing so will ease the frustration and make you feel more confident about your food choices and decisions.

Section 3
Never Diet, Again.

"The most important factors for a long life, I think, are partly in the genes; number two is lifestyle, which includes a healthy diet and regular exercise."
—John Gokongwei

Chapter 15
Healthy Eating as a Lifestyle

Now that you can separate fact from fad, have you started challenging some of your dieting beliefs?

Dieting is not how you should be living your life, nor the way you should be eating. You may be excited initially and follow the diet religiously, but eventually, you're going to relapse. The reason being is because you've heavily restricted yourself from eating foods within a specific food group and start building the urge to eat those foods again. Or you've placed so many restrictions on yourself (i.e., extreme calorie restriction and avoiding foods you love), which will make you feel the need to want to eat and enjoy your food freely.

Diets provide a short-term solution. They can get you quick results, which is what most people want. To live a healthy lifestyle requires a lot of effort, time, dedication, and patience – things that most people don't want to do.

How do you make healthy eating a lifestyle? Rather than focusing on what you can or cannot eat, focus on your habits and behaviors. Changing your habits and behaviors for the better will keep you grounded throughout your health journey and allow you to *stick* to eating well consistently and joyfully. After all, the best diet is the one you can maintain.

Here are my seven principles (not in order of importance) which will allow you to start making the shift from a restrictive diet to a lifestyle diet.

Principal #1 – Have the Right Mindset.

In my first book, *Fill Your Mind Before You Fill Your Plate*, I've mentioned the first pillar to living a healthier lifestyle is mindset. In my opinion, it all starts in the mind. You may think transitioning into a healthier lifestyle begins by signing up to a gym or seeing a nutritionist. While exercise and nutrition are important, you should focus first on your mind. You must practice self-discipline. Like a muscle that gets stronger as you exercise, you need to exercise and strengthen your willpower as the more you do this, the stronger your willpower will get.

Principal #2 – Be Patient.

Contrary to a diet which provides quick and easy fixes, adopting a healthy lifestyle needs time and patience. Don't set out on your healthy journey thinking that results will come easily or quickly. I'll tell you from now the journey is long, difficult and bumpy – but not impossible. For example, we know peak weight loss in lifestyle interventions occurs at around six months. Changing habits requires, on average, 66 days (not 21 days as often mentioned). It highlights a couple of reasons why time and patience are required to live a healthy lifestyle consistently.

Principal #3 – Put in the Effort.

Chase a healthy lifestyle, don't let it chase you. You are in the driver's seat. It's you who will take charge and make the decisions for yourself, not anybody else. Nothing comes easy in life, and living a healthy lifestyle is definitely not easy. You have to understand that it will be a difficult journey which will require a lot of effort. If it were effortless, we'd be living in a world full of fit and healthy people, wouldn't we?

Principal #4 – Consistency.

Consistency…consistency…consistency! All seven principles are key to living a healthier lifestyle, but I can't stress enough the importance of this one. With the abundance of information today, it's not necessarily a lack of education which is a barrier to people living healthier (although I'm still surprised at the lack of education in some people, given the level of awareness and information available). It's the implementation. It's the daily practice of eating well, exercising, and sleeping well. Consistency is the small but *daily* practice of healthy habits. That's right; consistency requires you to focus throughout each day, week, month and year. It requires effort all year long, regardless of whether it's summer or not.

The most important thing is just to show up, even if it's small practices every day. Too tired to exercise? Go for a ten-minute walk. Too lazy to cook food? Order from a healthy restaurant. Struggling to meditate for 10 minutes? Start by meditating for two minutes. By showing up every day and taking the right steps in your health journey, you'll slowly get to where you need to be and build stronger, better and more long-lasting habits – ultimately allowing you to become more consistent.

Principal #5 – Do What You Enjoy.

If you want to be consistent, and commit to the lifestyle, then do something you enjoy. Don't engage in physical activity you hate. Try out different classes and types of training styles, find the one you enjoy, and stick to it. When it comes to nutrition, don't diet! Diets aren't enjoyable. By having the freedom to eat the foods you love and enjoy (in a healthy manner, of course), you'll enjoy your life so much more and automatically find yourself making better food choices and decisions.

Principal #6 – Have Fun.

With enjoyment comes fun. Indeed, a healthy lifestyle needs to be a fun and exciting one. To have fun, practice balanced eating by following the 80–20 rule. Focus on eating clean, whole, unprocessed foods 80% of the time while eating the foods you crave and enjoy 20% of the time. This 20% is critical in helping propel you forward throughout your journey because it provides you with a sense of freedom and flexibility in the way you eat. In this 20%, eat the foods you love (chocolates, sweets, chips, biscuits, etc.), go out with family and friends to restaurants and have some dessert at a social gathering. Give in to your cravings from time to time, as eating foods which provide you with satisfaction will make you have fun with your food without feeling restricted. One thing to note is that the 80–20 rule is applied per week and not per day.

Principal #7 – Reward Yourself

A healthy lifestyle is all about celebrating the 'small wins.' If you've accomplished a smaller goal which has helped you take another step toward the bigger goal, reward yourself! Whether this comes through positive self-talk or rewarding yourself with a meal or food you love, the key is recognizing your achievements. Praise yourself, be proud of your work and effort, and commit to practicing healthy habits again as you work toward your next goal.

You may have noticed that I haven't told you which foods to eat or avoid, and I have not prescribed exercises for you to do. I'm focusing on behavioral qualities needed to help you focus on adopting a healthy lifestyle. There's no magic diet, and there's no superior way of eating or exercising. Through having control over your mind, patience, work ethic, consistency, enjoyment, fun, and celebrating small wins, you'll be on your way to making a healthy lifestyle your new normal. You'll achieve personal greatness and be the best and healthiest you can be.

"Shame is a soul eating emotion."
—Carl Gustav Jung

Chapter 16
Overcoming Food Guilt and Shame

How's your relationship with food?

Often, we link feelings of guilt and shame to food, leading to a poor relationship with food and yourself.

Food guilt is when you feel bad about a decision or behavior regarding food. It could be something you did or didn't do. It could be beating yourself up emotionally for eating a cookie when you feel you should not have or regretting not having that piece of cake with your coffee.

Food shame is when you judge yourself personally, stemming from something food related. It could be attacking yourself because of your lack of willpower to refuse the cookie, and therefore telling yourself that you just 'suck' at achieving your weight-loss goals.

We experience food shame and guilt because of this 'diet' culture. When you break the so-called rules or eat something which is not in line with the diet you're following, you'll feel guilty and shameful, hindering your relationship with food. You can also judge your worthiness and doubt yourself as a human being.

So how do you overcome food guilt and shame? Here are some tips:

Be easy on yourself. It's okay to mess up now and then. It's okay to 'break the rules' from time to time. If you ate a cookie or two, it's fine. If you had a slice of cake at a birthday party, it's fine. Be easy on yourself, accept the decision you made, and commit to getting back on track.

Don't diet. Dieting places you in a box with a label. There are so many limitations and restrictions that it invites feelings of guilt and shame when you step out of line.

Make it a lifestyle. When you make healthy eating a lifestyle, it helps ease the pressure, allowing you to eat more flexibly and feel comfortable mentally and emotionally. If you truly are healthy, you won't stress at all about eating.

Don't compare yourself with others. If your friend orders a salad, but you want a fried chicken burger, order the fried chicken burger. Enjoy and embrace the burger. When you don't compare yourself with others, you'll feel more at ease with yourself. Everyone has different goals, needs, wants, and desires. Do as you please and own your decisions without inviting any negative emotions (i.e., guilt and shame).

Have your own beliefs. The diet culture has inflicted many beliefs upon us, making us think that certain foods are bad and should be avoided, such as 'burgers are bad' or 'white rice is bad.' Have your own beliefs, and consider if they are factual or some arbitrary belief created by this diet culture.

Look at the bigger picture. What are you going to remember 2, 5, or 10 years from now? Are you going to remember eating that cookie before going to bed? Are you going to remember the slice of cake you had at the birthday party? No. You will remember going to the birthday party, hanging out with your friends, and enjoying yourself. Think of the moments and experiences you shared with other people rather than focusing on these small details, which, again, will only bring in feelings of guilt and shame. Look at the bigger picture in life.

What about the weekends? Do you find yourself doing really well during the week and 'messing' up with your eating on weekends? Does this make you feel guilty and shameful?

If this happens to you, it's okay! It happens to all of us. The weekend is a time to relax and enjoy our food and any social activities we have planned (which also revolve around food). Free time and social events can easily throw you off track.

There could be many reasons that may cause you to overeat on weekends, but the good news is you can manage that and still eat well. Here are some of my tips which the diet culture won't teach you to help you avoid overeating on the weekends.

Find balance. Let's revisit the 80/20 rule. Aim to eat healthily on weekends 80% of the time and give into your cravings 20% of the time. There's no need to eat healthily 100% of the time or eat unhealthily 100% of the time.

Don't wait for the weekend to indulge. Sometimes it's a better idea to enjoy your 'cheat meal' during the week. By doing so, you won't find the need to overindulge on the weekends turning a cheat meal into a cheat day(s). Try and avoid the mentality of completely letting go on weekends, and instead, enjoy the odd 'cheat meal' during the week.

Think of your hunger and fullness levels. Part of mindful eating is paying attention to your hunger levels before eating and your fullness levels after eating. On a scale of 1–

10, one being starving and 10 being nauseous from overeating, be mindful of your hunger levels so you can make better food choices and portion control. Ideally, you want to be at a hunger and fullness level of anywhere between 4–6 on the scale, which translates to being hungry (4), neutral (5), or satisfied (6). Approach the table hungry but not starving and eat until satisfied and not stuffed. Below is a hunger scale for you reference:

Hunger Level	Rating
Starving	1
Ravenous	2
Growling	3
Hungry	4
Neutral	5
Satisfied	6
Full	7
Stuffed	8
Bloated	9
Nauseous	10

Stay hydrated. Often, we may feel hungry or experience sugar cravings, but this does not mean a lack of food per se.

It probably means you're dehydrated. So aim to keep track of your water intake, especially over the weekend.

Focus on the feeling. Think of the last time you ate a cheat meal? Did you feel heavy, bloated, or uncomfortable? How do you feel after a healthy meal? I'm sure you felt light, happy and more at ease mentally, emotionally and physically. The next time you consider overeating, remind yourself of how you felt and commit to making a healthier decision the next time. By focusing on the feeling, you'll realize how good you feel when you eat well, and it'll motivate you to stay on the healthy track even on the weekend. Remembering how you felt after indulging in a heavy meal makes you reconsider your options the next time you face a situation where you could indulge in a similar meal.

Guilt and shame are negative emotions linked to food that ultimately may lead to poor eating habits. With that, let's look at habit change next.

"Change might not be fast and it isn't always easy. But with time and effort, almost any habit can be reshaped."
—Charles Duhigg

Chapter 17
Habit Change

Take a second and think about brushing your teeth every morning or washing your hands after using the bathroom. Do you put any effort into remembering to do these things, or does it happen automatically? Are you even present when carrying out these actions?

These are rhetorical questions because these actions have become so automatic that they are now habits.

This is the point I want you to reach with your nutrition. I want you to practice healthy habits to the point where eating healthily feels automatic. I want you to get to the point where it becomes your new normal, where it becomes your lifestyle.

All habits share similar qualities. Your habits are triggered by a cue, an event, or a situation. Habits are formed through constant repetition, which then makes them automatic. Unfortunately, another characteristic of habits is that they are hard to break.

To understand habits and how to break them, you should understand the four stages: cue, change, response, and result.

The cue is the trigger. It could be a situation, an event, or an emotion.

Change is the feeling we get after an action. Without a need for change, there is no reason for us to act. In the case of brushing your teeth in the morning, it's not the act of brushing your teeth that is the driving force; it's the feeling of a clean mouth. It's the change from bad breath to good breath.

The response is the action or thought of performing the 'habit' and, in this case, the habit was to brush your teeth.

Finally, the response leads to a reward. The end goal of every habit is the reward. You perform a particular habit because it leads you to the desired reward, which usually provides satisfaction. The cue triggers the change, which leads to a response and provides a reward. Given all of this, it's important to note that habits shouldn't be eliminated – they should be replaced.

So how do you break old habits and form new ones?

Firstly, focus on one habit at a time. If you try to change multiple habits at once, you're going to feel overwhelmed and go back to square one. Focus only on the most important habit for you to change and take the baby step approach, tackling only this habit.

I will share the journey of a client who was struggling with her high consumption of chocolate and soda. "What's your priority?" I asked her. "To reduce your consumption of chocolate or soda?"

"Reduce my consumption of chocolate," she said. Given this, I took her on a habit-changing journey which focused on her priority.

It's hard to let go of things you have been enjoying for a long time, so it would not be wise to expect her to decrease the intake of both sodas and chocolate at once. My advice was for her to put all her effort into focusing only on reducing her consumption of chocolate while continuing to drink sodas without reduction.

The focus was on reduction rather than going cold turkey and cutting chocolate completely; we gradually built her confidence by starting with one chocolate-free day each week. After two weeks, her confidence had grown, and she was able to increase her chocolate-free time to two days each week. It boosted her confidence enough to start considering three days, then four days, etc. During this process, she continued drinking her sodas regularly, by the way.

Through gradual and slow habitual change, she was confident and able to go weeks without eating much chocolate. It was a successful change, yet a change which involved several weeks of hard work, dedication and sacrifice. It was only at this point that, using the same process, we started working on reducing her soda consumption.

It's essential to be aware of your confidence levels before focusing on any habit you want to start working on and when considering focusing on a new habit. Before considering this, ask yourself, on a scale of 0–10, how confident are you?

0	Not going to happen
1–2	Slightly confident
3–4	Somewhat confident
5–6	Probably okay
7–8	Fairly confident
9–10	Completely confident

Being at a 7–8 could work, depending on your personality type, but ideally, you want to be at a nine to start working on a new habit or even before focusing on your next habit. It could take you two weeks to feel completely confident, and in other instances, it could take you two months. Remind yourself that the habit-change process takes time, so practice patience, and trust and embrace the process. By focusing on your priorities and tackling one habit at a time, your habit-change journey will be smoother, less frustrating, and more achievable.

After narrowing down your priorities, you need to identify the cue or trigger which causes the habit.

What makes you eat?

Don't confuse this with why you eat. They're two different things.

So let me ask you again, what makes you eat? Is there a specific situation, mood, or time of day which makes you want to eat?

Food triggers can cause overeating and eventually weight gain. Being oblivious to what makes you want to eat may very well make you consume large amounts of food and sometimes foods you may very well regret eating. Each of us has different eating triggers, and some might be more obvious than others. For some, it can be the thought of a pizza that makes them want to eat, while others do not even think of food to trigger their eating.

Most of us experience certain triggers which fuel our cravings, sending our nutrition into a total mess when acted on. That's why learning to recognize your eating triggers will help you figure out how to manage them better and ultimately eat more healthily.

Watch out for these common food triggers.

Certain places and actions can be a trigger, like sitting down in front of the TV. Have you ever found yourself sitting on the couch, turning on the TV and mindlessly munching on food? Whether it's the couch or the TV, these are potential triggers to make you eat. Environmental triggers like the office, driving in the car, or even sitting at home can also make you eat.

What if you were scrolling through Instagram and then came across a picture of a delicious burger and then ordered it. What's the trigger here? Instagram. Social media is undoubtedly a trigger we experience in today's world. Following food accounts on social media can trigger you to eat certain types of food.

The types of food you eat can also be considered a trigger. Sugary foods or beverages can trigger your desire to want to eat more sweets. Believe it or not, but exercise is also considered an eating trigger. For some, exercise increases their hunger levels; others think that they can eat whatever they want by exercising. If you experience an increase in hunger levels when exercising, don't worry because it's normal.

Triggers are all around us. By planning and being aware of trigger situations, you can successfully manage things like emotional and stress eating, which will help you achieve the first step in habit change.

Throughout your health journey, mistakes and slip-ups will happen. You may find that the trigger has reclaimed control of your eating. If this does happen, look back and understand what went wrong. The continual quest to identify your eating triggers will increase your chance of success.

Maintain a positive attitude and continue your efforts of wanting to live a healthier lifestyle.

Find an alternative to the initial action. Alternative actions can be as simple as reading a book, calling a friend, or working on a music playlist. Do something to distract yourself from doing what triggered your action in the first place. Once you've identified the trigger, you must have a backup plan. Similar to exercise and nutrition, do what works best for you, regardless of what the alternate action may be – as long as it does not involve food.

How can you avoid triggered eating with social media? Well, maybe unfollow accounts which post tempting pictures of food, or just avoid using social media at certain times of the day, especially when you're hungry.

If you think the couch is a trigger, change the environment in which you watch TV. If it's the TV which is the trigger, read a book or do something other than watching TV to avoid eating unnecessarily. If driving in your car is a trigger, don't drive past restaurants or cafés which tempt you or have a bottle of water in the car to stay hydrated and full.

Sometimes your home can be a trigger too. Easily accessible sweets and chocolates around the house can trigger you to eat them, even though you may not necessarily be physically hungry. If that's the case, implement the 3 Rs to manage your home environment.

You first need to **RECOGNIZE** the foods which will help you on your journey and the foods which will be an obstacle. Then, you need to **REMOVE** the foods that are an obstacle to your journey. Finally, you have to **REPLACE** the foods you removed with healthier options.

It's all about being observant – looking at what's in your kitchen, TV room, work desk and even your car. If you don't control your environment, your environment will control you, making your journey so much more difficult.

If eating specific foods trigger your sugar craving cycle, limit your consumption of refined sugars (which kickstarts the cycle) and replace them with protein and fiber-rich food (i.e., fruits, nuts, yogurt, or vegetables), which are known to reduce sugar cravings. Don't forget to drink water, as sugar cravings and hunger can result from dehydration and not necessarily a lack of or the 'need' for sugar. If you know exercise is an eating trigger, there's nothing wrong with preparing a light snack or meal to eat after your session. This way, you can ensure eating a healthy meal and enhancing muscle recovery post-exercise.

Lastly, the new habit needs to be repeated over and over and over again. You form new habits because of repetition, so the more you perform your new habit, the more it will become ingrained and the quicker it will develop. This circles back to the notion of being consistent, a key component to making healthy eating a lifestyle. The more repetition, the more consistency – it's a cycle.

One technique to change your habits is through 'habit stacking,' a term coined by James Clear, the author of *Atomic Habits*. This book is by far the best I've read on habit-change as Clear offers simple, concise and practical ways to replace old habits with newly formed positive ones.

Clear said, "One of the best ways to build a new habit is to identify a current habit you already do each day and then stack your new behavior on top. This is called habit stacking. Habit stacking is a special form of implementation intention.

Rather than pairing your new habit with a particular time and location, you pair it with a current habit."

The habit stacking formula is as follows:

"Before/After [CURRENT HABIT], I will [NEW HABIT]."

Below are some examples that Clear mentions in his book:

"After I pour my cup of coffee each morning, I will meditate for one minute."

"After I take off my work shoes, I will immediately change into my workout clothes."

From a nutrition perspective, here's how you can use the habit-stacking technique:

After I eat lunch, I'll have a piece of fruit (this could be a good idea for those who tend to eat dessert after lunch. Fruits are a good replacement for dessert).

After I brush my teeth, I'll drink 500ml of water.

As Clear mentions, "The reason habit stacking works so well is that your current habits are already built into your brain. You have patterns and behaviors that have been strengthened over the years. By linking your new habits to a cycle that is already built into your brain, you make it more likely that you'll stick to the new behavior. Once you have mastered this basic structure, you can begin to create larger stacks by chaining small habits together. This allows you to take advantage of the natural momentum that comes from one behavior leading into the next."

Habits are everything. There are so many factors that impact your success in living a healthier lifestyle, but let me tell you this, it's your habits which ultimately determine how consistent and successful you will be – for the long haul.

Replacing old habits with new, positive ones will lead to long-term and permanent change. So from now on, do the best you can to develop positive habits to be the healthiest you can be.

"Meaningful, long-lasting change doesn't happen overnight. Be patient with yourself, and know that the progress is in the process. Start by finding something you enjoy, and create space in your schedule to practice that thing each day. Make it a priority, and you will eventually make it a habit."
—Melissa Steginus

Chapter 18
Ten Healthy Habits

Now that you know more about habit change, I want to share my ten healthy habits for weight loss, sleeping better, moving more, reducing sugar cravings, snacking better and managing stress.

Ten Healthy Habits for Weight Loss:

1. **500 calorie deficit.** Whether through exercise, cutting back on food, or both, aim for a calorie deficit of 500 calories per day.
2. **Start with vegetables.** Whatever your meal, load up on vegetables before digging into the other components of the meals. The fiber in vegetables will help fill you up. In fact, this is a technique as part of the 'pre-loading' strategy. Pre-loading is essentially loading the stomach with fiber or water-rich foods or beverages, allowing you to feel full even before starting your main meal. By doing so, you'll be able to portion control better and eat less than you would have if you were not pre-loading. For example,

having a bowl of soup or salad, eating a fruit or two, or drinking 1–2 glasses of water before your meal will add to satiety, helping you eat less in your main meal.
3. **Catch some sleep.** At least 7–8 hours of sleep per night is crucial for weight loss. A lack of sleep can increase cortisol levels, the stress hormone, in the body. A rise in cortisol triggers your body to start saving the energy to allow you to push through your sleep-deprived day. This energy is stored as fat. Hence why proper sleep can positively impact your ability to lose weight from fat.
4. **Smaller plates.** Deceive your eye! Eating from a smaller plate makes your meal look bigger, even if the portions are the same.
5. **Exercise.** Run, walk, dance, bike, lift weights. Do whatever it takes to get that heart rate up for 30 minutes – One hour, five days a week. If you think you can do more, then gradually increase your exercise duration and frequency.
6. **Eat slowly.** It takes 20 minutes for your brain to register that you're full. Put your fork down between bites and savor your meal slowly. The slower you eat, the faster you'll feel full, making it less likely that you'll overeat.
7. **Hydrate, hydrate, hydrate.** Drink at least two liters of water per day. Sometimes, your brain tells you you're hungry when really, your body is just thirsty.
8. **Easy on the sugar.** Slowly wean yourself off sugar from teas, coffees, sodas, and juices. This added sugar is just empty calories and can hinder your weight loss.

9. **Increase protein intake.** You can burn calories simply by eating protein. Protein suppresses the appetite by increasing satiety and also reduces sugar cravings. Opting for high-protein meals will control your hunger levels throughout the day, allowing you to make the right food choices and portion control easier.
10. **Increase fruit intake.** Like protein, the fiber, vitamins and minerals found in fruit keep you feeling satisfied, suppress your appetite while also reducing sugar cravings.

Ten Healthy Habits to Move More:

1. **Start with 30 minutes.** If you're new to fitness, start with short exercise sessions, then gradually progress as you develop a routine and your body gets used to it. Start slowly; there's no need to kill yourself from the beginning. Focus on consistency rather than intensity, especially at the start.
2. **Standing desk.** If your work allows it, a standing desk can help improve your posture, burn more calories, and improve productivity.
3. **Make it fun.** By making your exercise fun and enjoyable, you'll want to exercise more. Find an activity you like, and stick to it.
4. **Find a workout partner.** It can be really motivating to workout with someone that shares your goals. It can be a friend or family member.

5. **Try out new exercises.** Looking to do yoga? Maybe you want to work on mobility or strength? Whatever it is, work on something new to keep your training fresh and exciting.
6. **Don't overdo it.** There's no need to kill yourself at every workout. It will lead to soreness, and you may need more rest days to recover. Again, think consistency over intensity.
7. **Social Media.** Check out fitness apps or follow trainers on social media for workout routines.
8. **Reward yourself.** Set small goals and reward yourself once you achieve them. This method keeps you motivated to exercise consistently.
9. **Consistency is key.** Going to the gym once a month is not going to cut it. Keep at it regularly, and you will see results.
10. **Organize your day around exercise.** Set a time every day to exercise. Doing this gives you a routine and prioritizes exercise.

Ten Healthy Habits for Sleeping Better:

1. **Set a sleep schedule.** Your body clock follows a routine. Set your sleep and wake-up time and stick to it.
2. **Temperature.** Keep the temperature between 18–20°C. The literature shows this to be the ideal temperature to fall and stay asleep.
3. **Keep 30 minutes for mindfulness.** Put your phone away at least 30 minutes before bed to wind down.

Try to read or stretch to get yourself ready for bed. If you can't start with 30 minutes, start with five minutes, then each week, increase the time by another five minutes until you reach 30 minutes, and ideally 60 minutes before bed without using your phone.
4. **Bedroom sleep makeover.** Block out any light with blackout curtains, and buy earplugs if you live in a noisy neighborhood. Your sleep environment highly impacts your sleep quality and quantity.
5. **Cut stimulants.** Avoid caffeinated beverages after 4 pm, as caffeine makes it difficult for you to fall asleep. Caffeine remains in the blood for 10 hours. Even if you are tolerant of caffeine, drinking caffeinated beverages close to bedtime could still disrupt your sleep.
6. **Avoid all technology.** Bright light stimulates your mind. Blue light from electronic devices can reduce the production of melatonin in the brain by 22%. Melatonin is a hormone released by the pineal gland at night and is responsible for our sleep-wake cycle. Avoid using any technology before bed.
7. **Bedtime bath.** Taking a relaxing, hot bath before bedtime can help you unwind and relax your mind and body.
8. **A glass of warm milk.** If you can tolerate dairy, why not opt for a glass of milk before bed? Tryptophan, an amino acid found in milk, can help you sleep better.
9. **Small meals in the evening.** Consuming a large meal close to bedtime can affect your sleep as your body

tries to digest the food. If you're hungry, stick to healthy and light snacks at night.
10. **Avoid sleep-aid.** As tempting as they sound, sleeping supplements and medication can cause daytime drowsiness and reliance. Try to improve sleep naturally if you can.

Ten Healthy Habits for Reducing Sugar Cravings:

1. **Rethink your drink.** If you're adding sugar or syrups to your tea or coffee, slowly cut them down. If you already drink black coffee or tea without any sugar, then well done. Keep your drinks simple, and aim to eat your calories instead of drinking them.
2. **Minimize cereals.** Limit your intake of sugary cereals, especially in the morning. Healthier alternatives such as oatmeal or even whole wheat cereals are a much better option.
3. **Slowly decrease your sweet consumption.** Cut out one sweet food from your nutrition plan each week. The more you do this, the less you'll need something sweet.
4. **Train your brain.** If you like to eat something sweet after main meals, try to reduce this indulgence; choose one meal a day when you'll avoid having something sweet afterward. It will help train your brain not to crave something sweet after a meal.

5. **Increase protein intake.** A high protein intake can make you feel full for longer and doesn't raise blood sugar levels as refined carbs and sugars do.
6. **Eat more fiber.** Increase fiber intake through fruits and vegetables. Fiber helps maintain blood sugar levels, thereby reducing sugar cravings.
7. **Drink more water.** Sometimes your body craves sugar not because you are hungry but because you're dehydrated. Drink water to stay hydrated and reduce sugar cravings.
8. **Healthy swaps.** Choose healthier sweet options. Rather than consuming sweets and chocolate, foods such as fruits, dried fruits, and flavored yogurt are healthier replacements. Choose dark chocolate instead of milk chocolate. Eat a protein bar instead of a chocolate bar. Nutrition is not eliminating – it's healthy swapping.
9. **Exercise.** Once you exercise, you'll subconsciously start changing the way you eat. By exercising, you'll begin to find yourself eating healthier and feeling better.
10. **Limit simple sugars.** It is easy to minimize simple sugars like brown sugar and honey. Even though honey may have amazing benefits, it is still a simple sugar.

Ten Healthy Habits for Snacking Better:

1. **Go nuts!** Nuts are packed with essential nutrients needed to keep you feeling fresh and alert during the

day. While nuts are healthy, they are high in calories, so don't go too nuts!
2. **Eat a combination of food.** There's no need to focus on one specific food group. You can combine fruit with healthy fats, like nuts or avocado. You can have a slice of toast with a piece of cheese or organic nut butter.
3. **Snack mindfully.** Just like you need to be mindful when eating a main meal, be mindful when snacking. A snack should literally be a snack. It is so easy to get carried away and mindlessly eat a lot of food, so snack mindfully.
4. **Make snacking easy.** Fruits like apples, bananas, and grapes are easy to take with you wherever you go. Nuts, protein bars, and light sandwiches are also easy-to-carry options for snacks. There's no need to overcomplicate snacks; keep them simple.
5. **Breakfast for snacks.** You can easily mimic breakfast foods as a snack. Why not try some mashed avocado on a slice of toast or a cup of Greek yogurt with some fruits?
6. **Eat your grains.** If you have a long day ahead, go for some grains for a sustained release of energy. Low-salted pretzels, tortilla chips, or even a small pot of oatmeal are good snack ideas.
7. **Try some vegetables or fruits with a dip.** It can really make eating vegetables and fruits fun to do. Try some baby carrots with hummus, celery with yogurt, or even sliced bell peppers with guacamole. For fruits, I love the combo of sliced red apple or a banana with organic peanut butter.

8. **Rethink your drink.** Snacking doesn't only mean eating; it can also mean drinking a beverage. Stick to smart snack beverages like unsweetened tea or coffee, low-fat milk, and of course, still or sparkling water.
9. **Snacks for cravings.** Rather than reaching out for some milk chocolate or sweets, why not snack on foods like dried fruits, a protein bar, or even dark chocolate as a way to satisfy your cravings healthily.
10. **Snack when you're hungry.** Be mindful of how hungry you are before reaching out for a snack. Eating out of boredom or any emotion can lead to consuming unnecessary calories, which can easily be avoided. If you're hungry, eat. If you're not hungry, there's no need to snack.

Ten Healthy Habits for Stressing Less:

1. **Positivity Journal.** Every morning, write down three things you're grateful for; start your day off in a good mood.
2. **Brain fuel.** Feed your brain with the right food; the impact on your stress levels throughout the day will be evident. There is a direct link between food quality and mental health. Berries, dark chocolate, oily fish, walnuts, and turmeric can boost brain power.
3. **Exercise.** Not only is physical activity important for fitness, but it also increases the release of feel-good hormones and lowers cortisol levels in the body.

4. **Sleep better.** A lack of sleep stimulates stress hormone production (cortisol), increases the production of the hunger hormone ghrelin, and decreases the production of the fullness hormone leptin. This process can lead to an increase in food cravings and calorie intake. Aim for 7–8 hours of sleep every night.
5. **Avoid added sugar.** Prevent energy slumps by avoiding added sugar in tea and coffee as well as the consumption of sweets and chocolate, all of which can increase cortisol levels. Stick to natural sugar like that found in fruit.
6. **Find something you enjoy, and do it every day.** Reading, yoga, drawing, or exercising; every day, do something for at least 30 minutes that makes you happy.
7. **Time-out.** It is crucial to have some 'me-time' every once in a while. Take some time off from the day for yourself. Even if it's for 10 minutes a day without any distraction, it can make a big difference. Reward yourself.
8. **Time-management.** Structure in your life can significantly reduce your stress levels. Find a routine which works for you and stick to it. Feeling organized and in control can help you reduce stress.
9. **Accept it.** It's inevitable that you may feel overwhelmed at times. Recognize that now and again, stress is normal, and stay calm and rational during stressful times.

10. **Laugh.** Laughter is the best medicine. Not only does it burn calories, but it also releases serotonin which can help you feel good.

"We're all so busy we don't make time to enjoy our lives, good company, and good food."

—John Torode

Chapter 19
Eating for a Busy Lifestyle

Do you lead a busy lifestyle? Are you constantly swamped with work which distracts you from eating well or leads you not to eat at all?

Today, we live in a fast-paced world with imminent deadlines and lots of stress. The combination of a busy working day and stress can most definitely affect the way you eat. To combat your stress, you may eat, which usually leads to comfort (unhealthy) food choices, or you might not eat at all. In both cases, a hectic lifestyle may negatively impact your food choices and decisions.

As a nutritionist working with busy people looking to improve their food choices during stressful times, I've come up with simple and easy tips to help your nutrition on hectic days. Let me provide you with a simple crash course on how to eat well during a busy day.

Plan Ahead. This is one of the most important and effective things you can do. If you're anticipating a busy working day, spend 5–10 minutes the night before (or the morning of) to understand what your day will look like so that you can plan accordingly.

Meal Prep. After planning your day, a good idea is to prepare your meals. Meal prepping can save you time, money and help you with weight loss as you can ensure the availability of healthy foods throughout the day. If you need to get up early, make a sandwich the night before and keep it refrigerated so you can take it with you the following morning without feeling rushed. If you have meetings lined up, bring some easy-to-carry snacks such as fruits and nuts. When cooking meals, cook enough to have several meals available to eat at your convenience. For example, grill 3–4 chicken breasts at a time, cut up vegetables and roast or bake them in the oven, and even cook a batch of rice, pasta, or quinoa all in one go. Meal planning can help you stay fueled and energized throughout the day while maintaining your healthy routine.

Stay hydrated. Be sure to drink water throughout the day. Water keeps you energized and focused; it also helps you stay full and reduces sugar cravings. If you suffer from headaches or migraines, water can help solve this problem. Have water bottles visible to remember to drink, or take a water bottle from home and use it as a tracking tool for how much water to drink. There are also many mobile apps available to help you track your water intake.

Be Mindful. When was the last time you enjoyed a quiet meal, without any distractions? If you can't remember, you're not alone. It's pretty hard to find the time to eat in silence without checking your phone, watching TV, or socializing with others. Sadly for many, eating on the go has become the norm. As a result, people are barely chewing their food and eating way too fast. The idea of mindful eating is to be present and fully focused on your meal. I always say mindful eating is healthy eating. What you eat, how you eat, your portions, and even understanding why you eat all play a significant part in your health and body goals.

Did you know the speed of eating is a contributor to obesity and weight gain? It's true; swallowing down your food and finishing a meal within five minutes can lead you to overeat and consume way more calories than you need. I'm sure you've heard this many times before, but it takes the brain 20 minutes to register that it's full. As you eat and drink and your stomach begins to fill up, the stretch receptors in the stomach are activated, sending satiety (fullness) signals to the brain via the vagus nerve, a nerve connecting the brain and stomach. As the food enters the small intestine, appetite hormones are released, sending more satiety signals to the brain.

This process takes approximately 20 minutes. Eating faster than this process may cause you to overeat without even realizing it. The more slowly you eat, the quicker you'll register that you feel full, allowing you to consume less food and ultimately fewer calories. If your goal is weight loss or simply to feel healthy, your eating speed can play a significant role in helping you achieve your health and body goals. Sometimes the simple things in nutrition can lead to the biggest changes.

Cook 3-ingredient meals. If you search '3 ingredient meals' on Google, you'll find so many results. Prepare quick 3-ingredient meals during the week, and save the fancy meals for the weekend when you have more time to cook. There are hundreds of quick and easy recipes to follow which will probably take less time to prepare than for a takeaway to arrive.

Use a slow cooker. Use a slow cooker for cooking in bulk. With your dinner cooking while you are at work, you'll have a hot meal waiting when you get home.

Pre-chop vegetables and freeze them. When you have a chance, pre-chop your fruits and vegetables and prepare 'soup,' 'stir fry,' or 'smoothie' packs and store them in the freezer, ready to use when you need them. Nutritionally, we know there are negligible differences between fresh and frozen produce. If you're on a tight budget (and schedule), opting for frozen fruits and vegetables is a good idea.

Plan eating out. If you are planning to eat out, try to plan what you're going to eat. Researching the menu in advance is a good strategy, as you can browse through it on your own time and make the right choices.

By managing your nutrition on stressful and busy days, you'll be able to live a healthy lifestyle more consistently and avoid the nutrition pitfalls that these days can bring. Sure, you're busy balancing between work, time for yourself, the gym, family and friends – but strive to manage your nutrition, so your health is not secondary in your life; make your health a priority. The key is to learn how to deal with your food choices from the start in all situations. The stressful and busy days will keep on coming, and if you don't learn how to manage your choices and decisions from the outset, you're going to dig a deeper hole for yourself and make it harder to eat well. On the contrary, if you put the time and effort into making better decisions for such situations, you'll improve and get better and better, so that the next time you face a busy or stressful period, you'd have learned how to cope. This preparation will spare you many unwanted calories and kilograms on the scale in the long run, with the added benefit of less stress.

"Moderation. Small helpings. Sample a little bit of everything. These are the secrets of happiness and good health."

—Julia Child

Chapter 20
Dine with Me

Today's busy and fast-paced world has changed the way we eat. We're eating more ready-made on-the-go food, ordering in, eating out, and eating fewer home-cooked meals. I'm writing this during the COVID-19 pandemic, and while many people are shifting back to home-cooked meals, they will revert to the 'easier options' once this is all over.

Pandemic aside, the rise of technology and food delivery platforms has made eating very convenient and highly accessible. Ordering food has never been easier. It literally can take two clicks and 20 minutes for your food to arrive at your door. I understand there are many benefits. Still, I also think our busy lifestyles, lack of patience, and accessibility of quick and unhealthy food options are why the prevalence of obese, overweight, and diabetic individuals is increasing worldwide, among many other reasons.

The world is getting busier, more competitive, and hence much more stressful. Eating out and ordering in is inevitable, and with the rise of cloud kitchens, the accessibility of food will only get easier and easier. The upside is the global trend toward health and wellness, which means an increase in the availability of healthy restaurants and cafés. While we live busy and stressful lifestyles, no matter the situation we face, we can still make a conscious effort to make better food choices.

I'm sure you love eating out – we all do. We enjoy good company and good food. There is no reason why you can't eat out healthily and still enjoy your time. As alluded to previously, part of mindful eating is to be fully aware of the quality of food you put into your body. Being present when looking at a menu and carefully considering what to eat makes a big difference.

Follow these eating out tips to make sure you stay on the healthy track:

Have your say. You can easily get pressured to eat at places you would rather avoid. If you want to make sure you stay on the healthy track, why not have your say with family and friends and pick places you know offer healthy food options. Speak up!

Research the menu in advance. I still do this before eating out and find it to be such a useful practice. By researching the menu in advance, you'll have the time to browse through every option and choose what best suits your needs. You'll avoid making an irrational and rushed decision when deciding at the restaurant.

Watch out for keywords. When going through the menu, pay attention to keywords to help you understand how they prepare the meal; this will indicate the healthier option. Avoid words like battered, fried, deep-fried, creamy, and crispy. Instead, look out for words such as grilled, roasted, baked, air-fried, and steamed.

Ask for a take-away box. When you order your meal, ask for a takeaway box. When your food arrives, place half the portion in the box for the next day. That way, you're less likely to overeat. Since the 1950s, restaurant portions have almost tripled, which means the calorie composition of the meals has tripled too!

Drinks add up. Eat your calories; try not to drink them. Sugary drinks add empty calories to your meal. You could easily consume an extra 300 calories by just having two drinks. Aim to drink still or sparkling water.

Share a meal. Splitting a meal with your family or friend means a smaller portion and lowering your calorie consumption.

Make simple substitutions. Simple substitutions like a salad for fries or grilled vegetables for starchy carbs (i.e., rice) will make a difference. It's all about the small changes.

Dressing on the side. Restaurant dressings are full of calories, sugar, and preservatives, more than you can imagine. Order your dressing on the side and be in control of how much you drizzle on your meal, sparing yourself many extra and unnecessary calories and sugar.

Eat an appetizer only. If you're not too hungry, order an appetizer. There's no need to consume extra calories by forcing yourself to eat a main meal.

Control the desserts. If you feel like having a sweet ending, it's okay to have some dessert. Try to control the portion or swap it with a healthier alternative. Why not split one dessert between two, or substitute a creamy or chocolate-based dessert with a fruit-based one instead, like apple crumble. Or simply have fruits instead of dessert.

Eat slowly. You already know the importance of eating slowly, and here it is again. Especially when eating out, you can easily be distracted by socializing with other people at your table. It's important to practice eating slowly to control how much you eat.

To live a healthy lifestyle means ordering food, going out with family and friends and enjoying meals with them. It's not about locking yourself at home and eating home-cooked meals *all* the time. While eating at home is the better option, you still want to enjoy life. With these tips, you now know how to enjoy these moments healthily. If you truly are healthy, you'll know how to eat well anytime, anywhere.

"I've never been on a diet, and never will."
—Paul Hollywood

Chapter 21
Conclusion: Ditch the Idea of Dieting

Weight is just a number, seriously! Everyone gets so hung up with the number on the scale, leading to many mental, emotional, and physical health issues.

As a nutritionist, I never determine progress purely by weight. Use the number on the scale as an indication, but it's more important to focus on what makes up your weight. To determine this, I recommend a body composition test before you start your weight-loss journey. Focus on *what* weight you want to lose rather than *how much* you want to lose. Essentially, you want to be losing weight from fat instead of muscle. A body composition measurement is vital to determine what your weight consists of. Having more data rather than simply a number on the scale puts you in a better position to understand your progress.

Aside from analyzing your body composition, cues like differences in your clothes or even listening to feedback from family and friends (maybe they're noticing differences in the way you look) are much more important indicators of progress than those measured purely by the number on the scale.

I know that many people use the number on the scale as a motivation to stay on the right track. My advice is to avoid weighing yourself regularly, and if you do, don't focus on it too much. Sometimes there will be no change, but that doesn't mean you're not losing fat per se. Depending on the type of exercise you do and your nutrition regimen, you may very well gain muscle and lose fat, which typically results in no change on the scale, or perhaps an increase on the scale.

While I talked about weight, you may have noticed that I never focused on it as a means to the end. Nor did I talk about healthy eating to look good per se. Instead, I mentioned eating well to improve your health and wellbeing from a mental, physical, and emotional perspective. I understand weight and appearance may be important to you, but this should not be your sole motivation. I urge you to focus on being healthy for the sake of your mind, body, and soul. Once you feel good from the inside, it will radiate on the outside. You'll have more energy, feel happier, vibrant and comfortable, and in turn, you'll glow with confidence and positivity – regardless of your shape, size, form, or weight. That's what it's all about – the feeling. I can't stress enough the importance of focusing on the *feeling* to motivate you to become your healthiest self and make healthy living a genuine lifestyle.

How are your focus and concentration levels? Do you have more energy during the day? Is your mood better? Is your sleep improving? Maybe you're experiencing fewer headaches throughout the day? Do you feel lighter and less bloated?

With today's social media overload, it's easy to associate nutrition with looks. However, when you focus inwards and take note of how you feel as a result of eating well and then appreciate and value this feeling, you'll be in a much better position to keep pushing forward toward your goals and eat well *consistently*. Consistency is a key principle to living a healthy lifestyle.

By now, you've realized how society has created a certain stigma around diets – always correlating them with 'less.' Similarly, people also associate weight loss with eating less.

I'm here to change your perception of weight loss. I hope to have helped you understand that weight loss does not necessarily mean depriving yourself and restricting the amount and types of food you eat.

Let me recap. You might think that significantly lowering your caloric intake will help you lose weight. While a calorie deficit is needed to lose weight, too big of a deficit can backfire. If you're burning a lot of calories and not giving your body enough to function optimally, your metabolism will slow down over time. If you go for an extended period in an extreme calorie deficit, your body will start producing and storing fat to protect your organs and help you survive this extreme calorie restriction. One of the benefits of fat is insulation, so with severe calorie cuts comes increased fat production and storage.

Your lifestyle and environment also play a big role in living a healthy lifestyle. Factors like exercise, sleep, and stress highly impact your ability to lose weight and achieve any health goal you set for yourself. At the same time, your habits will determine your success in achieving your goals;

therefore, it is key to learn how to form life-long habits to help you stay consistent throughout your journey.

Dieting can be quite toxic for many people. The lack of freedom and flexibility, feelings of restriction and limitation and a lack of enjoyment are the many reasons why diets don't work. The stigmatizing, restriction and labeling diets bring is not healthy. Foods are labeled as 'good' or 'bad,' refraining from eating certain foods or food groups, reaching a certain body weight, looking a certain way, and actions deemed 'right' or 'wrong' only place more of an emotional and mental strain on people. Yet, with all that, unfortunately, people are still dieting.

Throughout this book, I've mentioned that it's best to eat in a balanced and enjoyable way rather than a diet. Eating healthy as a lifestyle does not mean anti-healthy or anti-nutrition. You now know that you can eat well and make healthy food choices and decisions without the need to be hard on yourself. You can also eat foods you enjoy.

Weight loss does not equal food deprivation. You can still eat your meals and enjoy yourself while making sure you eat nutrient-dense foods to improve your health and well-being.

My purpose is to give you the tools and resources you need to empower you to live freely and make your own choices which are best for you and your body without putting too much pressure on yourself. Once you're comfortable in your own skin and in control of your choices, you will be consistent with your habits to ultimately eat healthy for the long term. This is when you've successfully followed the *lifestyle* diet.

Today more than any other time in history, we're constantly bombarded with information. Be it from social media, friends, family, influencers, or the internet; we're in an information overload which only makes us more confused. Again, a lot of this information comes from non-credible sources, and it reinforces the philosophy and approach evoked by the diet culture.

I have highlighted many ways in which you can avoid dieting and eat with flexibility and freedom. Here are a few other ways to avoid being consumed with the idea of dieting as the path to achieve your health, body, and nutrition goals.

Unfollow social media accounts. You already know by doing your due diligence, you can obtain information from credible sources. Do your research on people you follow, and if they don't seem credible enough, unfollow them.

Nourish your body. Eat foods you enjoy and those that are nutrient-dense to nourish your whole body.

Self-compassion. Speak kindly to yourself. There's no need to place yourself under unnecessary pressure.

Work with someone. In doing your due diligence, research people who also have an anti-diet approach to nutrition and work with them. They'll help you focus on eating better and improving your relationship with your food and yourself while creating positive eating habits to see long-term changes to your health.

Aside from these strategies, perhaps you can look into intuitive and mindful eating. Intuitive eating was created in 1995 by registered dietitians Evelyn Tribole and Elyse Resch. It's a way of eating which focuses on allowing your body to guide you on what and how much to eat and is based on ten core principles: be aware of your hunger levels, challenge the 'food police,' and be kind to yourself, to name a few.

Earlier in the book, I mentioned Judith Matz and her role in promoting the anti-diet culture. Here's what she has to say about intuitive eating:

"With intuitive eating, instead of eating from the outside in, instead of following rules from a diet, people learn to use their internal physical cues to decide when, what, and how much to eat." By destigmatizing food choices, intuitive eating steers you back into your own body. Most people have "gotten so used to eating what they should and shouldn't eat, what's 'good' and 'bad,' they've really lost touch with 'What do I want? What would satisfy me?"

There are some overlapping principles when it comes to mindful eating, but there are differences. Mindful eating is about being present in the moment while eating. It's about focusing on the way you eat (i.e., chewing more), eating without any distractions, eating slowly, being aware of the quality and quantity of food you eat, as well as being mindful of how hungry you feel when approaching a meal, and how full you feel upon finishing a meal. I'm a big proponent of mindful eating, and it culminates a big chunk of my approach when working 1:1 with clients.

Regardless of which approach you choose, they both allow you the flexibility to make your own choices and decisions – putting you in the driver's seat.

Don't underestimate the power of being in control of what and how you eat. It can have a massive impact on your health and wellbeing on all levels. Once you achieve this sense of liberation, it allows you to eat with enjoyment rather than fear, and it will enable you to *eat* rather than diet. Matz said, "Remember that we come into this world born knowing how to do this. Babies, when they're hungry, cry. So really, we're going back to the way we were born: Eating."

References

1/Abbasi J. Interest in the Ketogenic Diet Grows for Weight Loss and Type 2 Diabetes. *Jama*. 2018;319(3):215. doi: 10.1001/jama.2017.20639

2/Altomare R, Damiano G, Palumbo VD, *et al.,* Feeding the brain : the importance of nutrients for brain functions and health. *Journal of Nutrition and Internal Medicine*. 2017;19(3):243–247.

3/Anton SD, Gallagher J, Carey VJ, *et al.,* Diet type and changes in food cravings following weight loss: findings from the POUNDS LOST Trial. *Eat Weight Disord*. 2012;17(2):e101–e108. doi: 10.1007/BF03325333

4/Austin GL, Ogden LG, Hill JO. Trends in carbohydrate, fat, and protein intakes and association with energy intake in normal-weight, overweight, and obese individuals: 1971–2006. *Am J Clin Nutr*. 2011;93(4):836–843. doi: 10.3945/ajcn.110.000141

5/Barnosky AR, Hoddy KK, Unterman TG, Varady KA. Intermittent fasting vs. daily calorie restriction for type 2 diabetes prevention: a review of human findings. *Transl Res.* 2014;164(4):302–311. doi: 10.1016/j.trsl.2014.05.013

6/Beleslin B, Cirić J, Zarković M, Vujović S, Trbojević B, Drezgić M. Srp Arh Celok Lek. 2007;135(7–8):440–446. doi: 10.2298/sarh0708440b

7/Brockmeyer T, Holtforth MG, Bents H, Kämmerer A, Herzog W, Friederich H-C. Starvation and emotion regulation in anorexia nervosa. *Comprehensive Psychiatry.* 2012;53(5):496–501. doi: 10.1016/j.comppsych.2011.09.003

8/Bueno NB, de Melo IS, de Oliveira SL, da Rocha Ataide T. Very-low-carbohydrate ketogenic diet v. low-fat diet for long-term weight loss: a meta-analysis of randomised controlled trials. *Br J Nutr.* 2013;110(7):1178–1187. doi: 10.1017/S0007114513000548

9/Cecchini MA, Root DE, Rachunow JR, *et al.,* (2006) Chemical exposures at the world trade center: use of the hubbard sauna detoxification regimen to improve the health status of New York City rescue workers exposed to toxicants. *Townsend Lett* 273, 58–65.

10/Chang ML, Nowell A. How to make stone soup: Is the "Paleo diet" a missed opportunity for anthropologists? *Evol Anthropol.* 2016;25(5):228–231. doi: 10.1002/evan.21504

11/Cialdella-Kam L, Kulpins D, Manore MM. Vegetarian, Gluten-Free, and Energy Restricted Diets in Female Athletes.

Sports (Basel). 2016;4(4):50. Published 2016 Oct 21. doi: 10.3390/sports4040050

12/Dahl WJ, Stewart ML. Position of the Academy of Nutrition and Dietetics: Health Implications of Dietary Fiber. *J Acad Nutr Diet*. 2015;115(11):1861–1870. doi: 10.1016/j.jand.2015.09.003

13/de Souza RJ, Bray GA, Carey VJ, *et al.,* Effects of four weight-loss diets differing in fat, protein, and carbohydrate on fat mass, lean mass, visceral adipose tissue, and hepatic fat: results from the POUNDS LOST trial. *Am J Clin Nutr*. 2012;95(3):614–625. doi: 10.3945/ajcn.111.026328

14/den Besten G, van Eunen K, Groen AK, Venema K, Reijngoud DJ, Bakker BM. The role of short-chain fatty acids in the interplay between diet, gut microbiota, and host energy metabolism. *J Lipid Res.* 2013;54(9):2325–2340. doi: 10.1194/jlr.R036012

15/Diaper AM, Law FD, Melichar JK. Pharmacological strategies for detoxification. *Br J Clin Pharmacol*. 2014;77(2):302–314. doi: 10.1111/bcp.12245

16/Duan W, Mattson MP. Dietary restriction and 2-deoxyglucose administration improve behavioral outcome and reduce degeneration of dopaminergic neurons in models of Parkinson's disease. *J Neurosci Res*. 1999;57(2):195–206. doi: 10.1002/(SICI)1097-4547(19990715)57:2<195::AID-JNR5>3.0.CO;2-P

17/Faris MA, Kacimi S, Al-Kurd RA, *et al.,* Intermittent fasting during Ramadan attenuates proinflammatory cytokines and immune cells in healthy subjects. *Nutr Res.* 2012;32(12):947–955. doi: 10.1016/j.nutres.2012.06.021

18/Fildes A, Charlton J, Rudisill C, Littlejohns P, Prevost AT, Gulliford MC. Probability of an Obese Person Attaining Normal Body Weight: Cohort Study Using Electronic Health Records. *Am J Public Health.* 2015;105(9):e54–e59. doi: 10.2105/AJPH.2015.302773

19/Fung TC, Vuong HE, Luna CDG, *et al.,* Intestinal serotonin and fluoxetine exposure modulate bacterial colonization in the gut. *Nat Microbiol.* 2019;4(12):2064–2073. doi: 10.1038/s41564-019-0540-4

20/Geller AI, Shehab N, Weidle NJ, *et al.,* Emergency Department Visits for Adverse Events Related to Dietary Supplements. *N Engl J Med.* 2015;373(16):1531–1540. doi: 10.1056/NEJMsa1504267

21/Gibson AA, Seimon RV, Lee CM, *et al.,* Do ketogenic diets really suppress appetite? A systematic review and meta-analysis. *Obes Rev.* 2015;16(1):64–76. doi:10.1111/obr.12230

22/Halagappa VK, Guo Z, Pearson M, *et al.,* Intermittent fasting and caloric restriction ameliorate age-related behavioral deficits in the triple-transgenic mouse model of Alzheimer's disease. *Neurobiol Dis.* 2007;26(1):212–220. doi: 10.1016/j.nbd.2006.12.019

23/Hill P, Muir JG, Gibson PR. Controversies and Recent Developments of the Low-FODMAP Diet. *Gastroenterol Hepatol (N Y)*. 2017;13(1):36–45.

24/Hruby A, Hu FB. The Epidemiology of Obesity: A Big Picture. *Pharmacoeconomics*. 2015;33(7):673–689. doi: 10.1007/s40273-014-0243-x

25/Hu T, Mills KT, Yao L, *et al.,* Effects of low-carbohydrate diets versus low-fat diets on metabolic risk factors: a meta-analysis of randomized controlled clinical trials. *Am J Epidemiol*. 2012;176 Suppl 7(Suppl 7):S44–S54. doi: 10.1093/aje/kws264

26/Huang RY, Huang CC, Hu FB, Chavarro JE. Vegetarian Diets and Weight Reduction: a Meta-Analysis of Randomized Controlled Trials. *J Gen Intern Med*. 2016;31(1):109–116. doi: 10.1007/s11606-015-3390-7

27/Hunter P. The inflammation theory of disease. The growing realization that chronic inflammation is crucial in many diseases opens new avenues for treatment. *EMBO Rep*. 2012;13(11):968–970. doi: 10.1038/embor.2012.142

28/ISSN 0254–4725 Dietary protein quality FOOD AND FAO...
http://www.fao.org/ag/humannutrition/35978-02317b979a686a57aa4593304ffc17f06.pdf. Accessed July 7, 2020.

29/Jackson E, Shoemaker R, Larian N, Cassis L. Adipose Tissue as a Site of Toxin Accumulation [published correction appears in Compr Physiol. 2018 Jun 18;8(3):1251]. *Compr Physiol.* 2017;7(4):1085–1135. Published 2017 Sep 12. doi: 10.1002/cphy.c160038

30/Johnston BC, Kanters S, Bandayrel K, *et al.,* Comparison of weight loss among named diet programs in overweight and obese adults: a meta-analysis. *JAMA.* 2014;312(9):923–933. doi: 10.1001/jama.2014.10397

31/Johnstone AM. Fasting – the ultimate diet? *Obes Rev.* 2007;8(3):211–222. doi: 10.1111/j.1467-789X.2006.00266.x

32/Johnstone A. Fasting for weight loss: an effective strategy or latest dieting trend? *Int J Obes (Lond).* 2015;39(5):727–733. doi: 10.1038/ijo.2014.214

33/Kalm LM, Semba RD. They Starved So That Others Be Better Fed: Remembering Ancel Keys and the Minnesota Experiment. *The Journal of Nutrition.* 2005;135(6):1347–1352. doi: 10.1093/jn/135.6.1347

34/Kesavarapu K, Kang M, Shin JJ, Rothstein K. Yogi Detox Tea: A Potential Cause of Acute Liver Failure. *Case Rep Gastrointest Med.* 2017;2017:3540756. doi: 10.1155/2017/3540756

35/Kikuchi M, Ushida Y, Shiozawa H, *et al.,* Sulforaphane-rich broccoli sprout extract improves hepatic abnormalities in male subjects. *World J Gastroenterol.* 2015;21(43):12457–12467. doi: 10.3748/wjg.v21.i43.12457

36/Kim MJ, Hwang JH, Ko HJ, Na HB, Kim JH. Lemon detox diet reduced body fat, insulin resistance, and serum hs-CRP level without hematological changes in overweight Korean women. *Nutr Res.* 2015;35(5):409–420. doi: 10.1016/j.nutres.2015.04.001

37/Klein AV, Kiat H. Detox diets for toxin elimination and weight management: a critical review of the evidence. *J Hum Nutr Diet.* 2015;28(6):675–686.
doi: 10.1111/jhn.12286

38/Kracker M, *et al.,* The cadmium content of protein drinks and nutritional powders. *Journal of the Academy of Nutrition and Dietetics.* (2016)

39/La Merrill M, Emond C, Kim MJ, *et al.,* Toxicological function of adipose tissue: focus on persistent organic pollutants. *Environ Health Perspect.* 2013;121(2):162–169. doi: 10.1289/ehp.1205485

40/Last AR, Wilson SA. Low-carbohydrate diets. *Am Fam Physician.* 2006;73(11):1942–1948.

41/Levinson JA, Sarda V, Sonneville K, Calzo JP, Ambwani S, Austin SB. Diet Pill and Laxative Use for Weight Control and Subsequent Incident Eating Disorder in US Young Women: 2001–2016. *American Journal of Public Health.* 2020;110(1):109–111. doi: 10.2105/ajph.2019.305390

42/Luppino FS, de Wit LM, Bouvy PF, *et al.,* Overweight, obesity, and depression: a systematic review and meta-analysis of longitudinal studies. *Archives of general psychiatry.* https://www.ncbi.nlm.nih.gov/pubmed/20194822. Published March 2010. Accessed July 6, 2020.

43/Makkapati S, D'Agati VD, Balsam L. "Green Smoothie Cleanse" Causing Acute Oxalate Nephropathy. *Am J Kidney Dis.* 2018;71(2):281–286. doi: 10.1053/j.ajkd.2017.08.002

44/Manheimer EW, van Zuuren EJ, Fedorowicz Z, Pijl H. Paleolithic nutrition for metabolic syndrome: systematic review and meta-analysis. *Am J Clin Nutr.* 2015;102(4):922–932. doi: 10.3945/ajcn.115.113613

45/McRae MP. Health Benefits of Dietary Whole Grains: An Umbrella Review of Meta-analyses. *J Chiropr Med.* 2017;16(1):10–18. doi: 10.1016/j.jcm.2016.08.008

46/Metzgar M, Rideout TC, Fontes-Villalba M, Kuipers RS. The feasibility of a Paleolithic diet for low-income consumers. *Nutr Res.* 2011;31(6):444–451.
doi: 10.1016/j.nutres.2011.05.008

47/Neuvonen PJ. Clinical pharmacokinetics of oral activated charcoal in acute intoxications. *Clin Pharmacokinet.* 1982;7(6):465–489.
doi: 10.2165/00003088-198207060-00001

48/Obert J, Pearlman M, Obert L, Chapin S. Popular Weight Loss Strategies: a Review of Four Weight Loss Techniques. *Curr Gastroenterol Rep*. 2017;19(12):61. Published 2017 Nov 9. doi: 10.1007/s11894-017-0603-8

49/Park GD, Spector R, Goldberg MJ, Johnson GF. The expanded role of charcoal therapy in the poisoned and overdosed patient. *Arch Intern Med*. 1986;146(5):969–973.

50/Paoli A, Rubini A, Volek JS, Grimaldi KA. Beyond weight loss: a review of the therapeutic uses of very-low-carbohydrate (ketogenic) diets. *European journal of clinical nutrition*. https://www.ncbi.nlm.nih.gov/pubmed/23801097. Published August 2013. Accessed July 6, 2020.

51/Paoli A. Ketogenic diet for obesity: friend or foe? *International journal of environmental research and public health*. https://www.ncbi.nlm.nih.gov/pubmed/24557522/. Published February 19, 2014. Accessed July 6, 2020.

52/Polak R, Phillips EM, Campbell A. Legumes: Health Benefits and Culinary Approaches to Increase Intake. *Clin Diabetes*. 2015;33(4):198–205.
doi: 10.2337/diaclin.33.4.198

53/Rokholm B, Baker JL, Sorensen TI. The leveling off of the obesity epidemic since the year 1999 – a review of evidence and perspectives. *Obes Rev* 2010; 11: 835–846.

54/Sarris J, Logan AC, Akbaraly TN, *et al.,* Nutritional medicine as mainstream in psychiatry. *The Lancet.*

Psychiatry. https://www.ncbi.nlm.nih.gov/pubmed/26359904. Published March 2015. Accessed July 6, 2020.

55/Sarwar Gilani G, Estatira Sepehr, Protein Digestibility and Quality in Products Containing Antinutritional Factors Are Adversely Affected by Old Age in Rats, *The Journal of Nutrition*, Volume 133, Issue 1, January 2003, Pages 220–225, https://doi.org/10.1093/jn/133.1.220

56/Sarwar Gilani G, Wu Xiao C, Cockell KA. Impact of antinutritional factors in food proteins on the digestibility of protein and the bioavailability of amino acids and protein quality. *The British Journal of Nutrition*. https://www.ncbi.nlm.nih.gov/pubmed/23107545. Published August 2012. Accessed July 7, 2020.

57/Seid H, Rosenbaum M. Low Carbohydrate and Low-Fat Diets: What We Don't Know and Why We Should Know It. *Nutrients*. 2019;11(11):2749. Published 2019 Nov 12. doi: 10.3390/nu11112749

58/Shepherd SJ, Gibson PR. Nutritional inadequacies of the gluten-free diet in both recently-diagnosed and long-term patients with coeliac disease. *J Hum Nutr Diet*. 2013;26(4):349–358. doi: 10.1111/jhn.12018

59/Staudacher HM, Lomer MCE, Farquharson FM, *et al.*, A Diet Low in FODMAPs Reduces Symptoms in Patients With Irritable Bowel Syndrome and A Probiotic Restores

Bifidobacterium Species: A Randomized Controlled Trial. *Gastroenterology.* 2017;153(4):936–947. doi: 10.1053/j.gastro.2017.06.010

60/Susser ES, Lin SP. Schizophrenia after prenatal exposure to the Dutch Hunger Winter of 1944–1945. *Archives of general psychiatry.* https://www.ncbi.nlm.nih.gov/pubmed/1449385. Published December 1992. Accessed July 6, 2020.

61/Susser E, Neugebauer R, Hoek HW, *et al.,* Schizophrenia after prenatal famine. Further evidence. *Arch Gen Psychiatry.* 1996;53(1):25–31. doi: 10.1001/archpsyc.1996.01830010027005

62/SyndemicsTheLancet. https://www.thelancet.com/series/syndemics. Accessed July 6, 2020.

63/Tarantino G, Citro V, Finelli C. Hype or Reality: Should Patients with Metabolic Syndrome-related NAFLD be on the Hunter-Gatherer (Paleo) Diet to Decrease Morbidity? *J Gastrointestin Liver Dis.* 2015;24(3):359–368. doi: 10.15403/jgld.2014.1121.243.gta

64/Thorning TK, Raben A, Tholstrup T, Soedamah-Muthu SS, Givens I, Astrup A. Milk and dairy products: good or bad for human health? An assessment of the totality of scientific evidence. *Food Nutr Res.* 2016;60:32527. Published 2016 Nov 22. doi: 10.3402/fnr.v60.32527

65/Tinsley G, Urbina S, Santos E, *et al.,* A Purported Detoxification Supplement Does Not Improve Body Composition, Waist Circumference, Blood Markers, or Gastrointestinal Symptoms in Healthy Adult Females. *J Diet Suppl.*2019;16(6):649–658.
doi: 10.1080/19390211.2018.1472713

66/Varady KA. Intermittent versus daily calorie restriction: which diet regimen is more effective for weight loss? *Obes Rev.* 2011;12(7):e593-e601.
doi: 10.1111/j.1467-789X.2011.00873.x

67/Wilkinson DJ, Hossain T, Hill DS, *et al.,* Effects of leucine and its metabolite β-hydroxy-β-methylbutyrate on human skeletal muscle protein metabolism. *The Journal of physiology.*
https://www.ncbi.nlm.nih.gov/pmc/articles/PMC3690694/.
Published June 1, 2013. Accessed July 7, 2020.

68/Yu J, Marsh S, Hu J, Feng W, Wu C. The Pathogenesis of Nonalcoholic Fatty Liver Disease: Interplay between Diet, Gut Microbiota, and Genetic Background. *Gastroenterol Res Pract.* 2016;2016:2862173.
doi: 10.1155/2016/2862173

www.ingramcontent.com/pod-product-compliance
Lightning Source LLC
Chambersburg PA
CBHW040520220526
45473CB00013B/2931